LIPOCRINOLOGY
The Relationship between Lipids and Endocrine Function

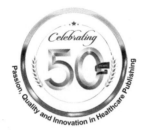

LIPOCRINOLOGY
The Relationship between Lipids and Endocrine Function

Editors

Sanjay Kalra MD DM
Consultant
Department of Endocrinology
Bharti Hospital
Karnal, Haryana, India

Gagan Priya MD DM
Senior Consultant
Department of Endocrinology
Fortis Hospital
Mohali, Punjab, India

Forewords
Brian Tomlinson
Ashwin B Mehta

JAYPEE BROTHERS MEDICAL PUBLISHERS
The Health Sciences Publisher
New Delhi | London | Panama

Jaypee Brothers Medical Publishers (P) Ltd

Headquarters

Jaypee Brothers Medical Publishers (P) Ltd
4838/24, Ansari Road, Daryaganj
New Delhi 110 002, India
Phone: +91-11-43574357
Fax: +91-11-43574314
Email: jaypee@jaypeebrothers.com

Overseas Offices

J.P. Medical Ltd
83 Victoria Street, London
SW1H 0HW (UK)
Phone: +44 20 3170 8910
Fax: +44 (0)20 3008 6180
Email: info@jpmedpub.com

Jaypee-Highlights Medical Publishers Inc
City of Knowledge, Bld. 235, 2nd Floor, Clayton
Panama City, Panama
Phone: +1 507-301-0496
Fax: +1 507-301-0499
Email: cservice@jphmedical.com

Jaypee Brothers Medical Publishers (P) Ltd
17/1-B Babar Road, Block-B, Shaymali
Mohammadpur, Dhaka-1207
Bangladesh
Mobile: +08801912003485
Email: jaypeedhaka@gmail.com

Jaypee Brothers Medical Publishers (P) Ltd
Bhotahity, Kathmandu, Nepal
Phone: +977-9741283608
Email: kathmandu@jaypeebrothers.com

Website: www.jaypeebrothers.com
Website: www.jaypeedigital.com

© 2019, Jaypee Brothers Medical Publishers

The views and opinions expressed in this book are solely those of the original contributor(s)/author(s) and do not necessarily represent those of editor(s) of the book.

All rights reserved. No part of this publication may be reproduced, stored or transmitted in any form or by any means, electronic, mechanical, photocopying, recording or otherwise, without the prior permission in writing of the publishers.

All brand names and product names used in this book are trade names, service marks, trademarks or registered trademarks of their respective owners. The publisher is not associated with any product or vendor mentioned in this book.

Medical knowledge and practice change constantly. This book is designed to provide accurate, authoritative information about the subject matter in question. However, readers are advised to check the most current information available on procedures included and check information from the manufacturer of each product to be administered, to verify the recommended dose, formula, method and duration of administration, adverse effects and contraindications. It is the responsibility of the practitioner to take all appropriate safety precautions. Neither the publisher nor the author(s)/editor(s) assume any liability for any injury and/or damage to persons or property arising from or related to use of material in this book.

This book is sold on the understanding that the publisher is not engaged in providing professional medical services. If such advice or services are required, the services of a competent medical professional should be sought.

Every effort has been made where necessary to contact holders of copyright to obtain permission to reproduce copyright material. If any have been inadvertently overlooked, the publisher will be pleased to make the necessary arrangements at the first opportunity. The **CD/DVD-ROM** (if any) provided in the sealed envelope with this book is complimentary and free of cost. **Not meant for sale.**

Inquiries for bulk sales may be solicited at: jaypee@jaypeebrothers.com

Lipocrinology: The Relationship between Lipids and Endocrine Function / Sanjay Kalra, Gagan Priya

First Edition: **2019**

ISBN: 978-93-5270-388-3

Printed at: Samrat Offset Pvt. Ltd.

Dedicated to

Our mentors
Late Professor A. C. Ammini
and
Professor Nikhil Tandon
who taught us the true meaning of patient centered care

Contributors

Editors

Sanjay Kalra MD DM
Consultant
Department of Endocrinology
Bharti Hospital
Karnal, Haryana, India

Gagan Priya MD DM
Senior Consultant
Department of Endocrinology
Fortis Hospital
Mohali, Punjab, India

Contributing Authors

Sameer Aggarwal MD DM
Consultant Endocrinologist
Head, Department of Endocrinology
Apex Plus Super-Speciality Hospital
Rohtak, Haryana, India

Jaikrit Bhutani MBBS
Post Graduate Junior Resident
Department of Medicine
Pandit Bhagwat Dayal Sharma Post Graduate
Institute of Medical Sciences
Rohtak, Haryana, India

Sambit Das MD DM PGD Endocrinology
Consultant Endocrinology
Apollo Centre for Obesity
Diabetes and Endocrinology, Apollo Hospitals
Bhubaneswar, Odisha, India

Ankush Desai MD DM
Consultant Endocrinology (Professor)
Department of Medicine
Goa Medical College
Bambolim, Goa, India

Emmy Grewal MD DM
Consultant Endocrinology
Department of Endocrinology
Ivy Hospital
Mohali, Punjab, India

Rajat Gupta MD DM
Consultant Endocrinologist
Department of Endocrinology
Alchemist Hospital
Panchkula, Haryana, India

Jubbin J Jacob MD DNB MNAMS
Professor and Head, Endocrine and
Diabetes Unit
Department of Medicine
Christian Medical College and Hospital
Ludhiana, Punjab, India

Arjin P Jacoby MD
Consultant Physician
Department of Medicine
Nav Jivan Hospital
Satbarwa, Jharkhand, India

Parjeet Kaur MD DM
Consultant
Department of Endocrinology and Diabetes
Medanta - The Medicity Hospital
Gurugram, Haryana, India

Sunil K Kota MD DNB
Consultant Endocrinologist
Diabetes and Endocare Clinic
Berhampur, Odisha, India

KVS Hari Kumar MD DNB
Professor, Department of Endocrinology
Army Hospital (R&R)
New Delhi, India

Om J Lakhani MD DNB
Consultant Endocrinologist
Department of Endocrinology
Zydus Hospital
Ahmedabad, Gujarat, India

Lalit K Meher MD
Dean and Principal
Government Medical College and Hospital
Balangir, Odisha, India

Sunil K Mishra MD DM
Associate Director
Department of Endocrinology and
Diabetology, Medanta - The Medicity
Gurgaon, Haryana, India

Lakshmana P Nandhini MD DM
Assistant Professor
Department of Endocrinology
St. John's Medical College
Bangalore, Karnataka, India

Neelam Pandey MD DM
Consultant Endocrinologist
Department of Endocrinology, Max Hospital
Gurgaon, Haryana, India

Subhodik Pramanik MD DM
Senior Resident
Department of Endocrinology
Institute of Post Graduate Medical Education
and Research
Kolkata, West Bengal, India

Jayaprakash Sahoo MD DM
Associate Professor
Department of Endocrinology
Jawaharlal Institute of Postgraduate Medical
Education and Research
Puducherry, India

Altamash Shaikh MD DM
Consultant Endocrinologist, Diabetologist,
and Physician, Saifee Hospital
Mumbai, Maharashtra, India

Yashpal Singh MD DNB DM
Professor, Department of Endocrinology
Command Hospital
Panchkula, Haryana, India

Foreword

The novel word lipocrinology, at first glance, conjures a vision of an esoteric, hyper-cerebral discipline, bordering the realms of science fantasy and fiction. Nothing, however, can be further from the truth.

Lipocrinology is a comprehensive coverage of the complex relationship between lipid health and endocrine function. Planned and prepared with scientific vigor and passionate zeal, this book is a unique compendium of knowledge. It covers physiological, clinical, and pharmacological aspects of lipidology in a lucid and systematic manner.

It is fascinating to see the way in which these difficult topics have been discussed and connected in a reader-friendly way. The combination (*connessione*) of scientific curiosity (*curiosita*) and experience (*dimostrazione*), coupled with elucidation of evidence based science (*scienza*) creates a literary work that reminds one of Leonardo da Vinci's philosophical principles.

The innovative concept of lipocrinology is defined and described, before detailing the impact of each endocrine axis upon lipid health. The role of the adipose tissue as an endocrine organ is elaborated upon, as is the relevance of the Asian lipophenotype and lipotoxicity in diabetes. Subsequently, the utility of lipid estimation in risk stratification and clinical decision-making is explored. Minute detail has been paid to the lipotropic and endocrine aspects of hormonal and lipid lowering management. The editors present the most current information in their book by including a chapter on the endocrine considerations of PCSK9 inhibition.

The book flows seamlessly—discussion on the basics of physiology and biochemistry, leads on to risk stratification and clinical decision making, followed by expansion of various clinical concepts. The theme of endovigilance in lipid disorders highlights the need to make endocrine assessment an integral part of lipidology. Chapters on basic and clinical topics are followed by a section on pharmacological management and its lipo-endocrine ramifications.

With the dyslipidemia pandemic showing no signs of abating, the need for such a book is greater than ever before. Its contents are relevant for health care professionals from all disciplines, including cardiology and internal medicine in addition to lipidology and endocrinology. Through this publication, I hope that we will be able to improve the lipid health of patients across the world.

Brian Tomlinson
Past-President, Asian-Pacific Society of Atherosclerosis and Vascular Diseases
Member, Asia Lipid Academy Steering Committee
Adjunct Professor and Former Chair Professor, Department of Medicine and Therapeutics
The Chinese University of Hong Kong
Hong Kong SAR, China

Foreword

As cardiologists, we focus on improving the cardiovascular health of our patients. At the same time, we are mindful of other vascular beds, and the need to ensure comprehensive vascular homeostasis. To do this, we practice a multifactorial approach, in conjunction with colleagues from endocrinology, neurology, nephrology, and internal medicine.

One aspect of metabolic care, which binds us together, is lipid health. Dyslipidemia is an important contributor to cardiovascular, cerebrovascular, and peripheral arterial morbidity (and mortality). Improvement in lipids is also shown to improve long-term outcomes, if appropriate therapy is used.

All lipids are not the same, however. Neither are all persons with dyslipidemia similar to each other. Varying etiologies and pathogenetic mechanisms contribute to different lipophenotypes, which in turn respond uniquely to various lipid-lowering strategies. Understanding of this heterogeneity allows the cardiologist, and other medical professional, to practice person-centered lipidology in an effective manner.

Dr Kalra and Dr Priya facilitate this process by editing a simple, yet comprehensive, and detailed, yet easily readable, book on lipocrinology. The subject matter of lipocrinology is the relationship between lipid homeostasis and endocrine function, as well as its implications on screening, monitoring and therapy.

This well laid out book is structured as three sections. Section 1 describes the impact of hormones on lipids, and the usage of lipophenotype in endocrine clinical practice. Section 2 covers the impact of adipose tissue/lipids on endocrine glands, while section 3 expands upon the endocrinotropic and lipotropic effects of various drugs.

This information is essential for the practising cardiologist, who increasingly deals with patients with multiple endocrine comorbidities. The concepts expounded in this book will help improve overall metabolic and endocrine management in cardiac patients. The knowledge contained in these pages will also facilitate timely and proper cross-disciplinary referral, thus leading to superior outcomes.

I, therefore, recommend this book to all the students and practitioners of cardiology, and its allied specialties.

Ashwin B Mehta MD FACC FISE FICP FSCAI
Director
Department of Cardiology
Jaslok Hospital and Research Centre
Mumbai, Maharashtra, India

Preface

Lipid health is an essential part of medical and metabolic health. Owned by all specialties, including cardiology, nephrology, neurology, endocrinology, and internal medicine, lipid health is gradually developing as a separate discipline. However, most discussion on lipids tends to focus on the cardiovascular implications of dyslipidemia, and ways to minimize it. Relatively less attention is paid to the root causes of lipid abnormalities.

This book, on lipocrinology, highlights the endocrine and metabolic aspects of lipid health. Expert authors explore the myriad relationships between endocrinology and lipidology, to create a colorful canvas of knowledge and information. The links between endocrinology and lipidology are discussed in a well laid out rubric. The central role of lipid estimation in risk stratification of cardiovascular disease, as well as its significance in diagnosing, differentiating, prognosticating, and planning therapy for endocrine disease is covered.

The impact of endocrine dysfunction on lipid health, the need for bidirectional screening when clinically indicated are reflected upon. The importance of monitoring lipid function while using endocrine therapy, and endocrine function with lipid lowering treatment is highlighted as well.

As the pandemic of endometabolic disease spreads, this book should have more and more relevance for health care professionals who work tirelessly to fight it. Readers will find this collection of chapters useful for both theoretical learning and clinical practice. Students, teachers, experts, and researchers from basic science as well as clinical disciplines are sure to find both information and insight from the book.

Sanjay Kalra
Gagan Priya

Acknowledgments

We attest to the continued contribution of our teachers, peers, and colleagues, all of whom have contributed to our understanding of lipocrinology.

We appreciate the dynamism and diligence of the editorial team at Jaypee Brothers Medical Publishers (P) Ltd. The team has worked hard to create a book with beauty, which should find admirers across the world.

We acknowledge the selfless support we have received from our families and friends; without them, we would not have been able to complete this task.

We acquiesce to Saraswati, the goddess of learning, for her grace and benevolence.

Contents

Section 1 Lipids in Endocrinology

1. **Lipocrinology: Definition and Domains** — 3
   Gagan Priya, Sanjay Kalra

2. **Lipo-health and Endocrine System: Thyroid, Parathyroid, and Pituitary** — 9
   Parjeet Kaur

3. **Lipo-health and the Endocrine System: Adrenals** — 19
   Gagan Priya, Emmy Grewal, Neelam Pandey

4. **Lipo-health and the Endocrine System: Reproductive System** — 30
   KVS Hari Kumar

5. **Lipo-health and the Endocrine System: Pancreas** — 38
   Arjin P Jacoby, Jubbin J Jacob

6. **Lipid-health as an Aid to Clinical Decision-making in Endocrinology** — 50
   Sanjay Kalra, Gagan Priya

7. **Dyslipidemia as a Risk Factor for Atherosclerotic Cardiovascular Disease in Endocrinology** — 60
   Subhodik Pramanik, Om J Lakhani

Section 2 Endocrine Aspects of Lipidology

8. **Adipose Tissue as an Endocrine Organ** — 73
   Lakshmana P Nandhini, Ankush Desai, Jayaprakash Sahoo

9. **Lipotoxicity and Diabetes Mellitus** — 87
   Sameer Aggarwal, Jaikrit Bhutani

10. **The Asian Lipophenotype** — 97
    Altamash Shaikh

11. **Lipodystrophies: Endocrine Effects** — 109
    Emmy Grewal, Rajat Gupta

12. **Endovigilance in Lipid Disorders** — 121
    Sunil K Kota, Sambit Das, Lalit K Meher

Section 3: Management Issues in Lipocrinology

13. **Lipid-lowering Drugs in the Management of Endocrinopathy** 137
    Om J Lakhani, Subhodik Pramanik

14. **Lipotropic Effects of Drugs Used in Endocrinology and Diabetes** 146
    Gagan Priya

15. **Endocrine Effects of Lipid-lowering Drugs** 160
    Yashpal Singh

16. **PCSK-9 Inhibitors: Endocrine Considerations** 172
    Sunil K Mishra, Sanjay Kalra, Gagan Priya

Index 183

SECTION 1

Lipids in Endocrinology

CHAPTER 1

Lipocrinology: Definition and Domains

Gagan Priya, Sanjay Kalra

> **ABSTRACT**
>
> There exists a close synchrony between the endocrine system, adipose tissue, and lipid metabolism. The novel concept of lipocrinology describes "the study of the inter-relationship between lipid metabolism and endocrine function in health and disease". Dyslipidemia is commonly seen in endocrine disorders and lipid abnormalities may point to underlying endocrine illness in general clinical practice. Since the prevalence of both lipid disorders and endocrine diseases is on the rise, it is prudent to understand the multifaceted relationship between lipid health and endocrine health. This chapter introduces the concept of lipocrinology, highlighting the myriad ways in which this inter-relationship between hormones and lipids is clinically relevant and important.

INTRODUCTION

The concept of "lipocrinology" was proposed by us to describe "the study of the inter-relationship between lipid metabolism and endocrine function in health and disease".[1] There exists a close synchrony between the endocrine system and lipid and lipoprotein metabolism, and this is reflected in both normal physiology and pathophysiological states.

Dyslipidemia is a common occurrence in clinical practice and accounts for greater than half the global burden of cardiovascular disease and has been attributed to cause over 4 million deaths per annum as per World Health Organization (WHO) 2002 report.[2] The prevalence of hypercholesterolemia was estimated to range from 3 to 53% in men and 4 to 40% in women in the WHO MONICA project that collected data from across 32 populations in 19 countries.[4] As per the Indian Council of Medical Research-India Diabetes Study (ICMR-INDIAB), there was a disturbingly high prevalence of dyslipidemia in individuals more than or equal to 20 years age in both rural and urban regions, with hypercholesterolemia in 13.9%, hypertriglyceridemia in 29.5%, reduced high-density lipoprotein cholesterol (HDL-C) in 72.3%, and increased low-density lipoprotein cholesterol (LDL-C) in 11.8%. As high as 79% individuals had abnormalities in at least one of the lipid parameters studied.[3]

Understandably, a significant amount of medical research and literature has been dedicated to the management of dyslipidemia and atherosclerosis and the reduction of cardiovascular risk. Statins have revolutionized the management of lipid disorders and several other classes of lipid-lowering drugs including fibrates, ezetimibe, bile acid sequestrants, and peroxisome proliferator-activated receptor alpha (PPARα) agonists have been added to the armamentarium. Proprotein convertase subtilisin/kexin type 9 (PCSK9) inhibitors are another novel class of lipid-lowering drugs which hold great promise for the future. Many of these drugs, including the currently available lipid-lowering drugs, have pleiotropic effects that include endocrine effects as well.

However, despite clear evidence that dyslipidemia is a major driver for comorbidity and mortality related to noncommunicable diseases, it remains an underdiagnosed and undertreated anomaly in both developed and developing countries. The awareness regarding hypercholesterolemia was seen in only 0–33% men and women in the WHO MONICA project. Moreover, only 50% of individuals who were receiving lipid-lowering drugs had attained target cholesterol levels.[4] Similar alarming data was gathered between 1998 and 2007 from eight high- and middle-income countries. The percentage of individuals with undiagnosed high cholesterol varied from 16% in United States to 78% in Thailand. Of those who were being treated, the percentage of individuals achieving target levels ranged from 4% in Germany to 58% in Mexico.[5] Several factors contribute to this—clinical inertia in diagnosis and management of dyslipidemia, suboptimal dosing, drug intolerance, and poor drug adherence. At the same time, inability to diagnose and address other conditions such as endocrine disorders that contribute to abnormal lipoprotein homeostasis may result in suboptimal control.

In recent times, the prevalence of both dyslipidemia and endocrine disorders is increasing due to genetic as well as environmental factors. This is likely to create greater challenges in the clinical management of lipid disorders as well as endocrinopathies. But at the same time, this is also expected to create new opportunities in furthering our understanding of the interface between endocrinology and metabolism and development of new therapeutic possibilities. Several newer drugs that have effects on lipid and glucose metabolism as well hormonal milieu are in development.

In such a scenario, there is a clear need to improve our understanding of endocrine system and lipid metabolism and how these work in tandem in the causation of noncommunicable diseases. Hence, the novel field of lipocrinology is not only relevant, but also the need of the hour.

LIPID METABOLISM: EFFECTS ON ENDOCRINE PHYSIOLOGY

Lipids play an essential role in the development and functioning of key endocrine organs. Lipids are the precursor molecules in the enzyme pathways leading to steroid hormone synthesis in several endocrine tissues, including adrenals and gonads. Intracellular lipid metabolites such as inositol triphosphate and diacylglycerol are essential second messengers involved in the cellular signaling pathways for a wide variety of hormones. Lipids are an important energy fuel for several energy-intensive processes including spermatogenesis and oogenesis. Additionally, several lipid-lowering drugs have been demonstrated to have endocrine effects other than lowering of lipid levels.

THE ADIPOSE TISSUE AS AN ENDOCRINE ORGAN

Adipose tissue, in its own merit, is now considered as a key endocrine organ that works in tandem with other endocrine organs such as the adrenals, gonads, pancreas, thyroid, and pituitary to regulate energy homeostasis, glucose and lipid metabolism, inflammation and endothelial functions. Adipose tissue dysfunction and lipotoxicity are increasingly recognized as a significant contributor to diabetes pathophysiology, including impairment of insulin secretion and insulin action. Lipotoxicity also forms the common link between diabetes and comorbid conditions such as cardiovascular disease and nonalcoholic fatty liver disease. Furthermore, genetic or acquired lipodystrophies are themselves associated with disturbances in endocrine functions.

THE ENDOCRINE EFFECTS ON LIPID METABOLISM

On the other end of the spectrum, all players of the endocrine system modulate the distribution and the differentiation of adipose tissue and regulate its functions. Diseases of the endocrine system, be they hormone deficiency states or hormone excess states, are associated with significant alterations in lipid metabolism that may manifest clinically as dyslipidemia. Indeed, detection of dyslipidemia in general practice merits detailed clinical assessment to exclude endocrinopathies as a secondary cause of dyslipidemia. Dyslipidemia is also the main contributing factor causing increased cardiovascular risk seen in several endocrine disorders and while it may be amenable to correction by adequate treatment of the underlying endocrinopathy, it may need to be addressed separately. Likewise, several drugs used in the management of endocrine diseases can have clinically meaningful effects on lipid parameters and adipose tissue health.

LIPOCRINOLOGY: A STEP TOWARD NEWER INSIGHTS

The subject of lipocrinology covers these varied aspects of the complex and multifaceted interplay between the endocrine system, adipose tissue, and lipid metabolism. The framework, as outlined in box 1 provides an improved understanding of the physiological links between hormones and metabolism, particularly lipid metabolism and the pathophysiological changes in various endocrine disease states. An understanding of these inter-relationships can improve clinical decision-making and management by improving vigilance for lipid disorders in the practice of endocrinology and endocrine disorders in the practice of lipidology. The concept is relevant to not just practicing endocrinologists, but also general physicians, internists, and cardiologists. This novel discipline has the potential to further research in both lipidology and endocrinology.

This book is dedicated to these aspects of lipocrinology. In the first section "Lipocrinology in Endocrinology", the contribution of various endocrine organs to

SECTION 1: Lipids in Endocrinology

> **BOX 1** **Lipocrinology: domains and scope**
>
> **Endocrinology in lipocrinology**
> - Physiological considerations:
>   - Hormones regulate adipose tissue distribution and function:
>   - Insulin, glucocorticoids, estrogen, androgens, and growth hormone
>   - Hormones regulate lipid metabolism:
>   - Insulin, thyroid hormones, glucocorticoids, growth hormone, estrogen, and testosterone.
>   - Age and gender differences in fat distribution and lipid parameters:
>   - Puberty—increase in free fat mass with only small increase in subcutaneous fat, decrease in total LDL and non-HDL cholesterol at puberty, decrease in HDL, and increase in triglycerides in boys
>   - Aging—increase in fat mass, especially visceral fat
>   - Premenopausal women have lower LDL-C and higher HDL-C than men
>   - Postmenopausal women have higher LDL-C, small dense LDL, and Lp(a)
> - Pathophysiological considerations:
>   - Abnormal adipose tissue distribution in endocrine disorders
>   - Visceral obesity in diabetes or polycystic ovary syndrome (PCOS)
>   - Central obesity with Cushingoid habitus in glucocorticoid excess states
>   - Dyslipidemia in hormone deficiency or excess states:
>   - Diabetic dyslipidemia
>   - Hypothyroidism (overt and subclinical)
>   - PCOS
>   - Cushing's syndrome
>   - Growth hormone deficiency
>   - Acromegaly
>   - Male hypogonadism.
> - Therapeutic considerations:
>   - Effect of endocrine drugs on lipid health:
>   - Worsen lipid health—oral contraceptives, depomedroxyprogesterone (DMPA), androgen deprivation therapy, mitotane, anabolic steroid misuse, and glucocorticoids.
>   - Improve lipid health—GLP1RA, DPP4i, pioglitazone, metformin, insulin, octreotide, L-thyroxine, bromocriptine, cabergoline, growth hormone, and ketoconazole
>   - Use of endocrine drugs in the management of lipid disorders:
>   - Thyromimetics
>   - Saroglitazar
>   - Ketoconazole for familial hypercholesterolemia
>
> **Lipocrinology in endocrinology**
> - Physiological considerations:
>   - Lipid as precursors in hormogenesis
>   - Lipids as second messengers in intracellular cell signaling
>   - Adipose tissue as regulator of energy homeostasis
>   - Adipose tissue as a secretory endocrine organ
>   - Adipose tissue involvement in enzyme pathways for hormones
> - Pathophysiological relationships:
>   - Obesity and adipose tissue dysfunction in endocrine disorders:
>   - Obesity, diabetes, PCOS, metabolic syndrome, and nonalcoholic fatty liver disease

Continued

CHAPTER 1: Lipocrinology: Definition and Domains

Continued

- Lipotoxicity:
  - Contribution to β-cell dysfunction and insulin resistance in diabetes, microvascular and macrovascular complications, and nonalcoholic fatty liver disease
- Lipodystrophies:
  - Insulin resistance and diabetes, secondary PCOS, male hypogonadism
- Dyslipidemia as a contributor to cardiovascular risk in endocrine diseases:
  - Diabetes, PCOS, growth hormone deficiency, acromegaly, Cushing's syndrome, and male hypogonadism
- Therapeutic considerations:
  - Endocrine effects of lipid-lowering drugs:
    - Statins increase risk of new onset diabetes and may worsen glycemic control
    - PCSK9 inhibitors increase fasting plasma glucose and HbA1c
    - Clofibrate can cause syndrome of inappropriate antidiuretic hormone secretion (SIADH)
  - Lipid-lowering drugs in treatment of endocrine disorders:
    - Fenofibrate in diabetic retinopathy
    - Statins improve bone mineral density
    - Statins improve erectile dysfunction
    - Cholestyramine as adjunctive treatment in hyperthyroidism
    - Clofibrate in diabetes insipidus
    - Colesevelam improves glycemic control in diabetes

Other management issues in lipocrinology
- Lipids as an aid to diagnosis of endocrinopathies:
  - Hypothyroidism, hypogonadism, acromegaly, diabetes, and PCOS
- Lipid vigilance in endocrine disorders:
  - Hypothyroidism, diabetes, obesity, and PCOS
- Lipids in clinical decision-making:
  - Cardiovascular risk stratification in diabetes, higher LDL-C as a factor when treating subclinical hypothyroidism
- Lipids to monitor endocrine therapy:
  - Cholesterol levels were used to monitor thyroid replacement prior to advent of immunoassays

LDL, low-density lipoprotein; LDL-C, low-density lipoprotein cholesterol; HDL, high-density lipoprotein; HDL-C, high-density lipoprotein cholesterol; Lp(a), lipoprotein(a); GLP1RA, glucagon-like peptide-1 receptors agonists; DPP4i, dipeptidyl peptidase-4 inhibitor; HbA1c, hemoglobin A1C.

lipid health and the pathogenesis of dyslipidemia in endocrine disease are discussed. The clinical utility of lipid parameters in diagnosis of endocrinopathies and their impact on the clinical course and prognosis of endocrinopathies is also considered. We also discuss the need for lipid vigilance in endocrine diseases. The second section "Endocrinology in Lipocrinology" is dedicated to the role of the adipose tissue as an endocrine organ, the role of lipotoxicity in diabetes, and the Asian lipophenotype, endocrine aspects of lipodystrophies, and endocrine vigilance in lipid disorders. The final section focuses on "Management Issues in Lipocrinology" and elaborates upon the effects of lipid-lowering drugs in management of endocrinopathies, lipotropic effects of drugs used in endocrinology and diabetes, and endocrine effects of lipid-lowering drugs including *PCSK9* inhibitors.

We hope this book sensitizes the readers to a greater understanding of lipocrinology and inspires further research.

REFERENCES

1. Kalra S, Priya G. Lipocrinology – the relationship between lipids and endocrine function. Drugs Context. 2018;7:212514.
2. World Health Organization. Quantifying selected major risks to health. The World Health Report 2002. Reducing Risks, Promoting Healthy Life. Geneva: World Health Organization; 2002:47-97.
3. Joshi SR, Anjana RM, Deepa M, et al. ICMR-INDIAB Collaborative Study Group. Prevalence of dyslipidemia in urban and rural India: the ICMR-INDIAB study. PLoS One. 2014;9(5):e96808.
4. Tolonen H, Keil U, Ferrario M, et al. WHO MONICA Project. Prevalence, awareness and treatment of hypercholesterolaemia in 32 populations: results from the WHO MONICA Project. Int J Epidemiol. 2005;34(1):181-92.
5. Roth GA, Fihn SD, Mokdad AH, et al. High total serum cholesterol, medication coverage and therapeutic control: an analysis of national health examination survey data from eight countries. Bull World Health Organ. 2011;89(2):92-101.

Lipo-health and Endocrine System: Thyroid, Parathyroid, and Pituitary

Parjeet Kaur

ABSTRACT

There is a close relationship between lipid physiology and the endocrine system. Hormones regulate lipid metabolism and endocrine disorders are often associated with abnormalities in lipid parameters and cardiovascular risk. Hypothyroidism has been established as a secondary cause of dyslipidemia and it is related with increased total and low-density lipoprotein (LDL) cholesterol and increased risk for atherosclerotic cardiovascular disease. Thyroid hormones control the expression of LDL receptor by various means and increase reverse cholesterol transport. The increased total and LDL cholesterol observed in patients with hypothyroidism improves with levothyroxine therapy. While parathyroid hormone also has some effects on lipid metabolism, the changes in lipid parameters in individuals with hyperparathyroidism have been less consistently reported. Pituitary hormones regulate the function of downstream endocrine organs including thyroid, adrenals, and gonads. Growth hormone increases lipolysis and free fatty release, lipid mobilization and oxidation. Acromegaly is associated with hypertriglyceridemia and reduced high-density lipoprotein (HDL) cholesterol levels and these improve with treatment. Dyslipidemia related to growth hormone deficiency is primarily related to increased visceral adiposity and insulin resistance and amenable to treatment with growth hormone.

INTRODUCTION

Endocrine disorders can affect lipid metabolism and alter the plasma lipid levels, which may increase the risk of cardiovascular diseases. It is to be noted that the literature may not always be consistent in describing the alterations in lipid metabolism and plasma lipid and lipoprotein levels induced by endocrine disorders with several studies showing inconsistent results. Number of confounding factors can explain these differences such as the disease severity and duration, different ethnic populations, dietary factors, or coexisting obesity or diabetes. In this chapter,

SECTION 1: Lipids in Endocrinology

we have described the classical alterations in lipids associated with thyroid, parathyroid, and pituitary disorders that have been most consistently reported. Among the pituitary hormones, effect of growth hormone and prolactin on lipids has been discussed. Lipid disorders associated with cortisol and gonadal hormone alterations are discussed in relevant chapters.

THYROID HORMONE AND LIPIDS

A connection between hypothyroidism and lipid disorders has been documented since 1930s.[1] Indeed, serum cholesterol measurement was considered as a marker of hypothyroidism before radio-immunoassays were developed for serum thyroxine (T4), tri-iodothyronine (T3) and thyroid-stimulating hormone (TSH). In 1960s, Bastenie suggested an association between hypothyroidism and the advance of coronary heart disease (CHD) for the first time.[2]

Thyroid hormones are key regulators of lipid and lipoprotein metabolism. They upregulate the expression of the hepatic low-density lipoprotein (LDL) receptor and increase the clearance of LDL particles. This process is mediated via direct influence of thyroid hormone (TH) on the TH responsive elements in the promoter region of LDL receptor gene and through their effect on sterol regulatory element-binding protein-2 (SREBP-2).[1] Thyroid hormones also reduce the activity of proprotein convertase subtilisin-kexin type 9 (PCSK9), additionally increasing LDL clearance. While THs increase cholesterol biosynthesis by increasing the activity of 3-hydroxy-3-methylglutaryl-coenzyme A (HMG-CoA) reductase which drives the conversion of HMG-CoA to mevalonate, LDL oxidation and apolipoprotein B (apo B) synthesis is reduced.[3] Thyroid hormones have a positive influence on high-density lipoprotein (HDL) metabolism and raise reverse cholesterol transport by stimulation of hepatic lipase (HL) and cholesteryl ester transfer protein (CETP).[1] Triglycerides (TGs) may be reduced by their effect to increase apo A5. The lipotropic effects of THs are depicted in figure 1.

Lipid Abnormalities in Overt Hypothyroidism

The lipid profile of several overt hypothyroid patients is characterized by an increase in total and LDL cholesterol (LDL-C) levels.[3] The Influence of hypothyroidism on HDL cholesterol (HDL-C) and TGs is inconstant with either no change or a modest increase in levels.[4,5] High serum concentrations of apo A1 and apo B are also found in many hypothyroid patients.[6] O'Brien et al. studied 295 patients with overt hypothyroidism, 56% had Fredrickson type IIa dyslipidemia (hypercholesterolemia), 34% had type IIb (hypercholesterolemia and hypertriglyceridemia), 1.5% had type IV (hypertriglyceridemia) and 8.5% had no dyslipidemia.[7] In general, lipid abnormalities brought by hypothyroidism are pro-atherogenic and are more marked with severe hypothyroidism and restoration of thyroid function often leads to improvement of lipid profile. In addition to abnormal lipid concentrations, diastolic hypertension as well as abnormalities in endothelial function and C-reactive protein are additional contributing factors for the increased risk of CHD among patients with overt hypothyroidism.

CHAPTER 2: Lipo-health and Endocrine System: Thyroid, Parathyroid, and Pituitary

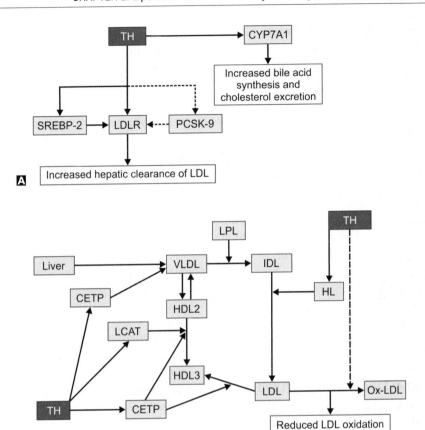

CETP, cholesteryl ester transfer protein; CYP7A1, cholesterol 7α-hydroxylase; HDL, high-density lipoprotein; IDL, intermediate-density lipoprotein; LCAT, lecithin cholesterol acyltransferase; LDL, low-density lipoprotein; LDLR, low-density lipoprotein receptor; LPL, lipoprotein lipase; Ox-LDL, oxidized low-density lipoprotein; PCSK-9, proprotein convertase subtilisin/kexin type 9; SREBP-2, sterol regulatory element-binding protein; TH, thyroid hormone; VLDL, very low-density lipoprotein.

FIG. 1: Lipotropic effects of thyroid hormone. **A,** Thyroid hormone (T3) upregulates the expression of low-density lipoprotein (LDL) receptors in liver by several mechanisms. It acts directly via thyroid responsive elements on the promoter region of the LDL receptor gene and stimulates its expression. It also increases the levels of sterol regulatory element binding protein-2 to further upregulate LDL receptor expression. In addition, T3 reduces the expression of proprotein convertase subtilisin/kexin type 9 (PCSK9) that is involved in LDL receptor degradation. Reduced PCSK9 activity results in increased LDL receptor levels. The net result is an increase in LDL clearance and reduction in LDL cholesterol levels. Thyroid hormone also stimulates bile acid synthesis and cholesterol catabolism by upregulation of 7 α-hydroxylase enzyme, that is a rate limiting enzyme in bile acid synthesis; **B,** Thyroid hormone increases the activity of cholesteryl ester transfer protein and lecithin/cholesterol acyltransferase, resulting in increased clearance of cholesteryl esters via high-density lipoprotein (HDL). The resultant increase in reverse cholesterol transport further contributes to the lipid-lowering effects of thyroid hormones. Hepatic lipase activity is also increased, leading to increased conversion of HDL 2 to HDL 3 and intermediate density lipoprotein to LDL. Thyroid hormone also increases LDL receptor expression in peripheral tissues and inhibits LDL oxidation.

Lipid Abnormalities in Subclinical Hypothyroidism

Most patients with subclinical hypothyroidism (SCH) have normal lipid profile. However, some have marginally high serum total and LDL-C, TGs and lipoprotein (a) (Lp-a) levels. In a unique study, the effect of SCH on total and LDL-C was greater in older (60–69 years) patients.[8] Ethnicity, duration of thyroid dysfunction and the occurrence of other metabolic abnormalities such as insulin resistance influence the impact of SCH on lipids. Subclinical hypothyroid patients with elevated TSH levels (>10 mIU/L) are more likely to show aberrations in lipid and lipoprotein levels.[9] The effects of T4 (levothyroxine) treatment on LDL-C in patients with SCH have been varying with some studies showing possibly beneficial changes and further studies showing no change.[10] The influence of T4 may be more prominent in those with overt hypercholesterolemia; in one study, serum LDL-C fell by 36 mg/dL (p <0.01) in such patients.[11] Serum HDL-C concentrations are low or normal in patients with SCH with a variable response to T4 therapy. In a meta-analysis, serum HDL-C did not increase significantly with T4 therapy.[12] Similarly, the effects of T4 treatment on serum Lp-a concentration in these patients are variable. Subclinical hypothyroidism may cause a very little difference in cardiovascular risk chiefly in young patients and patients whose TSH is more than 7–10 mIU/L.[13]

Lipid abnormalities seen in subclinical and overt hypothyroidism are summarized in table 1.

Mechanism for the Change in Lipid Parameters in Hypothyroidism
Low-density Lipoprotein Cholesterol

Thyroid hormone increases the expression of LDL receptors. The key mechanism for high LDL-C levels in hypothyroidism is decrease in the number of hepatic LDL receptors, resulting in diminished catabolism of LDL.[14] A reduction in LDL receptor activity has also been described. Thyroid hormone stimulates LDL receptor expression by increasing SREBP-2 and/or by direct effects on the LDL receptor promoter.[15] Raised PCSK9 levels in hypothyroidism result in decreased hepatic LDL receptor expression by reduction of LDL receptors. Also, action of TH on bile acids (BA) has been recently known as a separate hypocholesterolemic effect.[16] Bile acid synthesis can be affected by TH by increasing the action of a rate-limiting enzyme cholesterol

TABLE 1 Effect of hypothyroidism on lipids

Serum lipid parameter	Subclinical hypothyroidism	Overt hypothyroidism
Total cholesterol	Normal to increased	Increased
High-density lipoprotein cholesterol	No change	Normal to increased
Low-density lipoprotein cholesterol	Normal to increased	Increased
Triglycerides	Normal to increased	Normal to increased
Lipoprotein (a)	No change	Increased
Apolipoprotein B	Increased	Increased
Apolipoprotein A1	No change	Increased

7α-hydroxylase (CYP7A1), cholesterol catabolic enzyme, further reducing the plasma cholesterol levels. It is known that in hypothyroid patients a reduction in BA synthesis may cause increase in LDL-C levels. Several other known mechanisms of TH on lipid metabolism include—stimulation of expression of ABCG5 and ABCG8 transporters which facilitate the movement of cholesterol from the hepatocyte into the bile and reduce apo B production. Finally, hypothyroidism is also known to increase intestinal cholesterol absorption by its positive increase in Niemann-Pick C1-Like 1 (NPC1L1) intracellular cholesterol transporter.[18]

Triglycerides

Reduced lipoprotein lipase (LPL) activity, is responsible for the development of hypertriglyceridemia in hypothyroidism. Many studies have shown that TH stimulates LPL activity.[19] Additional mechanisms by which TH decreases TG levels include—stimulation of expression of apo A5, which potentiates the activity of LPL and decrease in angiopoietin-like protein 3, an inhibitor of LPL.[20] Lastly, hypothyroidism increases hepatic very-low density lipoprotein-triglyceride (VLDL-TG) secretion rate, which could also contribute to elevations in plasma TGs.

High-density Lipoprotein Cholesterol

Several key proteins involved in HDL metabolism and reverse cholesterol transport are regulated by TH. Activity of CETP, HL, lecithin cholesterol acyltransferase (LCAT), and scavenger receptor class B type 1 (SR-B1) are increased by TH and are decreased in hypothyroidism.[21] Hepatic lipase is also involved in the conversion of intermediate, density lipoproteins (IDL) to LDL. Its reduced activity in hypothyroidism has been related with the accrual of remnant-like particles in the serum of hypothyroid patients, contributing to cardiovascular risk.

The scope of TH replacement in patients with hypothyroidism and positive effect of lipid profile is discussed further in the chapter "Lipotropic effects of drugs used in endocrinology and diabetes". Specific agonists of thyroid hormone receptor subtype beta have the potential to reduce lipid levels without systemic effects of TH (17). The role of these thyromimetics as potential lipid-lowering drugs in also discussed in the same chapter.[17]

Effect of Hyperthyroidism on Lipids

Changes in lipid metabolism in patients with hyperthyroidism are generally opposite to those described for hypothyroidism. Effect of hyperthyroidism on lipids are summarized in table 2.

PARATHYROID HORMONE AND LIPIDS

Parathyroid hormone (PTH) also has well-defined effects on lipid metabolism additional to its actions on classic target organs. It activates hormone-sensitive lipolysis in adipose tissue by an adenylate cyclase mechanism.[22] Administration of parathyroid extract in canine and human subjects increases serum free fatty acids (FFA). Effect of primary and secondary hyperparathyroidism on serum lipids however is conflicting.

SECTION 1: Lipids in Endocrinology

TABLE 2 Effect of hyperthyroidism on lipids

Serum lipid parameter	Hyperthyroidism
Total cholesterol	Decrease
High-density lipoprotein cholesterol	Decrease
Low-density lipoprotein cholesterol	Decrease
Triglycerides	Variable
Lipoprotein (a)	Decrease
Apolipoprotein B	Decrease
Apolipoprotein A1	Decrease

Some studies have shown a reduction in serum cholesterol and TG concentrations in primary hyperparathyroidism (PHPT) and these normalized after parathyroidectomy (PTx).[23] Apparently, an increase in the incidence of type 4 hyperlipidemia in PHPT has also been reported with improvement after PTx.[24] Few studies have reported no change in serum lipids in longstanding hyperparathyroidism.[25] In a study of 86 PHPT patients, serum TG levels were significantly higher than the controls. Serum HDL-C, LDL-C, apo A and B were similar between the groups. After parathyroidectomy, while all lipoprotein values reduced significantly during short-term observation period, only serum TG remained diminished over long-term.[26] In an observational case-control study, mixed dyslipidemia, with high TG, HDL-C, and LDL-C predominated in low-risk asymptomatic persons, though only high LDL-C prevailed in symptomatic PHPT.[27] In a population-based study, PHPT was characterized by decreased HDL-C, increased total and VLDL-TGs and increased VLDL-C. Parathyroidectomy, with or without additive hormone replacement therapy in postmenopausal women, normalized the dyslipidemia.[28]

Secondary hyperparathyroidism (SHPT) and elevated serum PTH levels likely plays a permissive role for the progress of hyperlipemia in chronic kidney disease (CKD), characterized by elevated serum levels of TGs and LDL-C and low HDL-C. Hyperlipemia in CKD is caused by PTH-independent mechanisms, but is increased by the presence of SHPT. Changes in the action of insulin on lipolytic enzymes, perhaps mediated via increased levels of PTH, have been suggested to play an influential role.[29] In uremic patients with SHPT, some studies reported that PTx was not associated with an improvement of lipid disturbances; some reported a decrease in serum TG while others were unable to correlate serum PTH and TG concentration.

Taken together, data obtained in patients with PHPT and SHPT show that PTH exerts a deleterious effect on lipid metabolism especially TGs.

GROWTH HORMONE AND LIPIDS

The dominant effect of growth hormone (GH) on lipid metabolism is stimulation of lipolysis and lipid oxidation. The primary effect of GH in the basal state is to promote lipid mobilization and oxidation–these actions may be viewed as a means of switching substrate metabolism from glucose and protein utilization to lipid oxidation. Secretory pattern of GH plays an important role in the diurnal supply of fuel substrates. Nocturnal GH peaks precede the early morning rise of FFA by 2 hours.[30] Single exogenous GH pulse leads to marked increase in circulating levels of FFA and ketone bodies, reflecting stimulation of lipolysis and ketogenesis.[31] There is no evidence that GH acutely affects rate of TG synthesis.

Growth hormone suppresses LPL activity in human adipose tissue.[32] Growth hormone, probably via insulin-like growth factor 1 (IGF-1), also inhibits the conversion of cortisone to cortisol in adipose tissue from the abdomen by inhibiting the expression and activity of 11 β-hydroxysteroid dehydrogenase-1 (11β-HSD1). Reduced 11β-HSD1 expression and activity with reduced cortisol levels protect against central obesity via mechanisms that may involve reduced LPL activity, reduced differentiation of preadipocytes to mature adipocytes, and induction of a more favorable profile of anti-inflammatory adipokines.[33]

Acromegaly

Lipid abnormalities found in acromegaly, a GH excess state are summarized in table 3. In patients with acromegaly, frequently observed changes in lipids are increase in TGs and decrease in HDL-C. An increase in small dense LDL and apo B levels may be seen.[34] In patients with acromegaly, a positive correlation between GH and Lp-a levels, as well as the decrease of Lp-a after either medical or surgical treatment, indicate that Lp-a synthesis may be GH-regulated.[35]

Mechanism for Lipid Alterations in Acromegaly

Growth hormone excess can directly inhibit LPL activity and stimulate liver LDL-receptor expression, independent of IGF-1 levels.[36] The GH effect is probably displayed in the catabolism of LDL sub-fractions, because GH has been reported to induce hepatic LDL receptors, which will selectively lower LDL-2 more than LDL-3.[37] Several abnormalities in HDL lipid composition in patients with acromegaly are due to an impaired plasma LCAT action and a decreased phospholipid transfer protein. Plasma cholesterol esterification and cholesteryl ester transfer decrease with impaired reverse cholesterol transport, thereby leading to increased cardiovascular risk.[38] The increase in plasma TGs has been linked with increased TG production rate.[39] The LPL activity is also decreased in patients with acromegaly, which could decrease the clearance of triglyceride-rich lipoproteins.[40] Furthermore, insulin

TABLE 3 Effect of acromegaly on lipids

Serum lipid parameter	Acromegaly
Total cholesterol	Variable
High-density lipoprotein cholesterol	Decrease
Low-density lipoprotein cholesterol	Variable
Triglycerides	Increase
Lipoprotein (a)	Increase

SECTION 1: Lipids in Endocrinology

resistance and abnormal glucose metabolism that frequently occurs in patients with acromegaly likely contributes to abnormalities in TG metabolism.

Changes in lipoprotein metabolism are reversed after treating acromegaly either medically or surgically. Details of treatment effects are discussed in separate chapter.

Growth Hormone Deficiency

Hallmarks of adult-onset GH deficiency (GHD) include visceral obesity and impaired physical fitness, and result from a combination of prolonged GHD—lack of lipolytic and protein anabolic effects, and the underlying disease and its treatment, all of which translates into a state resembling metabolic syndrome. There is increased FFA flux from visceral fat. Dyslipidemia of GHD is characterized by elevation of total and LDL cholesterol and TGs with decreased HDL-C.[41,42] These abnormalities reverse on starting of GH therapy as detailed in another chapter.[43]

Mechanism for Lipid Alterations in Growth Hormone Deficiency

The increase in total and LDL cholesterol in GHD is likely due to a decrease in hepatic LDL receptors.[44] Increase in plasma TGs is due to increase in hepatic VLDL production and a reduction in VLDL clearance.[45]

PROLACTIN AND LIPIDS

Most studies have reported that patients with a prolactinoma have mildly increased total and LDL cholesterol while HDL-C is either decreased or unchanged.[46] Some studies have reported mild increase in TGs as well.[47] The mechanisms causing alterations in plasma lipid levels are not clear, but number of factors have been implicated. Prolactin may have direct effects on lipid metabolism as it decreases LPL activity in human adipose tissue. Plasma LPL activity is indeed decreased in patients with prolactinomas.[46,48] Increased prolactin levels are associated with decreased estrogen levels in women, which in turn can lead to elevated LDL and decreased HDL-C levels. Furthermore, obesity associated with high prolactin levels could adversely affect plasma lipid levels. Finally, suppression of GH secretion with large prolactinomas can result in abnormal plasma lipid levels.

CONCLUSION

Thyroid hormones are important regulators of lipid metabolism. Overt hypothyroid patients have increased serum total and LDL cholesterol levels. High serum TGs, IDL, apo A1, and apo B concentrations are also seen in many patients. Patients with SCH whose TSH concentrations are more than or equal to 10 mIU/L also have similar lipid finding. Hyperthyroidism, on the other hand, is associated with lower levels of total, LDL, and HDL cholesterol.

Growth hormone also mediates significant effects on lipid metabolism. In the basal state, the effect of GH is to promote lipid mobilization and oxidation. In acromegaly, increased Lp-a and TGs and reduced HDL are seen, and these improve with treatment. Growth hormone deficiency causes visceral obesity and insulin resistance, which reverses after initiating growth hormone replacement.

REFERENCES

1. Duntas LH, Brenta G. The effect of thyroid disorders on lipid levels and metabolism. Med Clin North Am. 2012;96(2):269-81.
2. Bastenie PA, Vanhaelst L, Neve P. Coronary-artery disease in hypothyroidism. Lancet. 1967;2:1221-2.
3. Lithell H, Boberg J, Hellsing K, et al. Serum lipoprotein and apolipoprotein concentrations and tissue lipoprotein-lipase activity in overt and subclinical hypothyroidism: The effect of substitution therapy. Eur J Clin Invest 1981;11:3-10.
4. Nikkila E, Kekki M. Plasma triglyceride metabolism in thyroid disease. J Clin Invest. 1972;51:2103-14.
5. Agdeppa D, Macaron C, Mallik T, et al. Plasma high density lipoprotein cholesterol in thyroid disease. J Clin Endocrinol Metab. 1979;49:726-9.
6. de Bruin TW, van Barlingen H, van Linde-Sibenius Trip M, et al. Lipoprotein(a) and apolipoprotein B plasma concentrations in hypothyroid, euthyroid, and hyperthyroid subjects. J Clin Endocrinol Metab 1993;76:121-6.
7. O'Brien T, Dinneen SF, O'Brien PC, et al. Hyperlipidemia in patients with primary and secondary hypothyroidism. Mayo Clin Proc. 1993;68:860-6.
8. Zhao M, Yang T, Chen L, et al. Subclinical hypothyroidism might worsen the effects of aging on serum lipid profiles: A population-based case-control study. Thyroid. 2015;25:485-93.
9. Wiersinga WM. Adult Hypothyroidism. In: LJ De Groot, Editors. Endotext [Internet]. South Dartmouth (MA): MDText.com, Inc.; 2000.
10. Rugge JB, Bougatsos C, Chou R. Screening and treatment of thyroid dysfunction: an evidence review for the U.S. Preventive Services Task Force. Ann Intern Med. 2015;162(1):35-45.
11. Michalopoulou G, Alevizaki M, Piperingos G, et al. High serum cholesterol levels in persons with 'high-normal' TSH levels: Should one extend the definition of subclinical hypothyroidism? Eur J Endocrinol 1998; 138:141-5.
12. Danese MD, Ladenson PW, Meinert CL, et al. Clinical review 115: Effect of thyroxine therapy on serum lipoproteins in patients with mild thyroid failure: a quantitative review of the literature. J Clin Endocrinol Metab. 2000;85:2993-3001.
13. Rodondi N, den Elzen WP, Bauer DC, et al. Subclinical hypothyroidism and the risk of coronary heart disease and mortality. JAMA, 2010;304(12):1365-74.
14. Thompson GR, Soutar AK, Spengel FA, et al. Defects of receptor-mediated low density lipoprotein catabolism in homozygous familial hypercholesterolemia and hypothyroidism in vivo. Proc Natl Acad Sci U S A 1981; 78:2591-5.
15. Shin DJ, Osborne TF. Thyroid hormone regulation and cholesterol metabolism are connected through sterol regulatory element-binding protein-2 (SREBP-2). J Biol Chem. 2003;278(36):34114-8.
16. Bonde Y, Breuer O, Lütjohann D, et al. Thyroid hormone reduces PCSK9 and stimulates bile acid synthesis in humans. J Lipid Res. 2014;55(11):2408-15.
17. Lin JZ, Martagón AJ, Hsueh WA, et al. Thyroid hormone receptor agonists reduce serum cholesterol independent of the LDL receptor. Endocrinology. 2012;153(12):6136-44.
18. Gälman C, Bonde Y, Matasconi M, et al. Dramatically increased intestinal absorption of cholesterol following hypophysectomy is normalized by thyroid hormone. Gastroenterology. 2008;134(4): 1127-36.
19. Kuusi T, Taskinen MR, Nikkila EA. Lipoproteins, lipolytic enzymes, and hormonal status in hypothyroid women at different levels of substitution. J Clin Endocrinol Metab. 1988;66(1):51-6.
20. Fugier C, Tousaint JJ, Prieur X, et al. The lipoprotein lipase inhibitor ANGPTL3 is negatively regulated by thyroid hormone. J Biol Chem. 2006;281(17):11553-9.
21. Tan KC, Shiu SW, Kung AW. Effect of thyroid dysfunction on high-density lipoprotein subfraction metabolism: Roles of hepatic lipase and cholesteryl ester transfer protein. J Clin Endocrinol Metab. 1998;83(8):2921-4.
22. Werner S, Löw H. Stimulation of lipolysis and calcium accumulation by parathyroid hormone in rat adipose tissue after adrenalectomy and administration of high doses of cortisone acetate. Horm Metab. Res. 1973;5:292-6.
23. Christensson T, Einarsson K. Serum lipids before and after parathyroidectomy in patients with primary hyperparathyroidism. Clin Chim Acta. 1977;78:411-5.
24. Ljunghall S, Lithell H, Vessby B. et al. Glucose and lipoprotein metabolism in primary hyperparathyroidism. Effects of parathyroidectomy. Acta Endocrinol (Copenh). 1978;89:508-89.

25. Vaziri ND, Wellikson L, Gwinup G, et al. Lipid fractions in primary hyperparathyroidism before and after surgical cure. Acta Endocrinol (Copenh). 1983;102:539-42.
26. Lacour B, Roullet JB, Liagre AM, et al. Serum lipoprotein disturbances in primary and secondary hyperparathyroidism and effects of para-thyroidectomy. Am J Kidney Dis. 1986;8:422-9.
27. Procopio M, Barale M, Bertaina S, et al. Cardiovascular risk and metabolic syndrome in primary hyperparathyroidism and their correlation to different clinical forms. Endocrine. 2014;47:581-9.
28. Hagström E, Lundgren E, Lithell H, et al. Normalized dyslipidaemia after parathyroidectomy in mild primary hyperparathyroidism: Population-based study over five years. Clinical Endocrinology. 2002;56:253-60.
29. Massry SG, Akmal M. Lipid abnormalities, renal failure, and parathyroid hormone. Am J Med. 1989;87(5N):42N-4N.
30. Rosenthal MJ, Woodside WF. Nocturnal regulation of free fatty acids in healthy young and elderly men. Metabolism. 1988;37:645-8
31. Moller N, Jorgensen JO, Schmitz O, et al. Effects of a growth hormone pulse on total and forearm substrate fluxes in humans. Am J Physiol. 1990;258:E86-91.
32. Richelsen B. Effect of growth hormone on adipose tissue and skeletal muscle lipoprotein lipase activity in humans. J Endocrinol Invest. 1999;22:10-5.
33. Moore JS, Monson JP, Kaltsas G, et al. Modulation of 11beta- hydroxysteroid dehydrogenase isozymes by growth hormone and insulin-like growth factor: In vivo and in vitro studies. J Clin Endocrinol Metab. 1999;84:4172-7.
34. Nikkila EA, Pelkonen R. Serum lipids in acromegaly. Metabolism. 1975;24(7):829-38.
35. Wildbrett J, Hanefeld M, Fucker K, et al. Anomalies of lipoprotein pattern and fibrinolysis in acromegalic patients: Relation to growth hormone levels and insulin-like growth factor I. Exp Clin Endocrinol Diabetes. 1997;105:331-5.
36. Rudling M, Olivecrona H, Eggertsen G, et al. Regulation of rat hepatic low density lipoprotein receptors. In vivo stimulation by growth hormone is not mediated by insulin-like growth factor I. J Clin Invest. 1996;97:292-9.
37. Rudling M, Norstedt G, Olivecrona H, et al. Importance of growth hormone for the induction of hepatic low density lipoprotein receptors. Proc Natl Acad Sci USA. 1992;89:6983-7.
38. Beentjes JA, van Tol A, Sluiter WJ, et al. Low plasma lecithin: cholesterol acyltransferase and lipid transfer protein activities in growth hormone deficient and acromegalic men: Role in altered high density lipoproteins. Atherosclerosis. 2000;153:491-8.
39. Christ ER et al. Effects of growth hormone (GH) replacement therapy on very low density lipoprotein apolipoprotein B100 kinetics in patients with adult GH deficiency: a stable isotope study. J Clin Endocrinol Metab, 1999. 84(1): p. 307-16.
40. Murase T, Yamada N, Ohsawa N, et al., Decline of postheparin plasma lipoprotein lipase in acromegalic patients. Metabolism. 1980;29(7):666-72.
41. de Boer H, Blok GJ, Voerman HJ, et al. Serum lipid levels in growth hormone-deficient men. Metabolism. 1994;43(2):199-203.
42. Abdu TA, Neary R, Elhadd TA, et al. Coronary risk in growth hormone deficient hypopituitary adults: increased predicted risk is due largely to lipid profile abnormalities. Clin Endocrinol (Oxf). 2001;55(2):209-16.
43. Norrelund H, Vahl N, Juul A, et al. Continuation of growth hormone (GH) therapy in GH-deficient patients during transition from childhood to adulthood: impact on insulin sensitivity and substrate metabolism. J Clin Endocrinol Metab. 2000;85:1912-7.
44. Parini P, Angelin B, Lobie PE, et al. Growth hormone specifically stimulates the expression of low density lipoprotein receptors in human hepatoma cells. Endocrinology. 1995;136(9):3767-73.
45. Moller N, Jorgensen JO. Effects of growth hormone on glucose, lipid, and protein metabolism in human subjects. Endocr Rev. 2009;30(2):152-77.
46. Pelkonen R, Nikkila EA, Grahne B. Serum lipids, postheparin plasma lipase activities and glucose tolerance in patients with prolactinoma. Clin Endocrinol (Oxf). 1982;16(4):383-90.
47. Heshmati HM, Turpin G, de Gennes JL. Chronic hyperprolactinemia and plasma lipids in women. Klin Wochenschr. 1987;65(11):516-9.
48. Ling C, Svensson L, Odén B, et al. Identification of functional prolactin (PRL) receptor gene expression: PRL inhibits lipoprotein lipase activity in human white adipose tissue. J Clin Endocrinol Metab. 2003;88(4):1804-8.

CHAPTER 3

Lipo-health and the Endocrine System: Adrenals

Gagan Priya, Emmy Grewal, Neelam Pandey

ABSTRACT

The adrenal glands have a high lipid content and cholesterol serves as a precursor for adrenal steroid hormones. At the same time, adrenal hormones regulate adipose tissue function and lipids. Glucocorticoids are key regulators of energy metabolism and affect lipid and lipoprotein metabolism through several mechanisms. Cushing's syndrome is associated with increased visceral and upper body fat, increased lipogenesis as well as increased lipolysis. The resultant changes in serum lipids include increase in total and low-density lipoprotein (LDL) cholesterol and triglycerides. In addition, patients with chronic glucocorticoid excess also have abnormal glucose metabolism, central obesity, hypertension, hypercoagulability, and endothelial dysfunction. Cardiovascular (CV) risk and mortality are significantly elevated, even after remission of hypercortisolism. This calls for aggressive multifactorial risk factor management with therapy targeted at optimization of glycemic control, blood pressure and lipids, and lifestyle modification, in addition to management of Cushing's syndrome. The effect of aldosterone, adrenal androgens, and catecholamines on lipid physiology, however, is not clearly understood. Lipid content of adrenal lesions can provide important clues in differentiating benign adenomas from malignant lesions in radiological imaging studies.

INTRODUCTION

The endocrine and lipid physiology are closely interlinked at several levels. Lipids modulate the function of endocrine organs and act as precursors for steroid hormone synthesis, and as second messengers in hormone signaling pathways. At the same time, endocrine function determines adipose tissue distribution and function, lipid metabolism, and overall metabolic health. Dyslipidemia is often seen associated with disorders of the endocrine system and modulates the risk of long-term cardiovascular (CV) complications that contribute toward morbidity and mortality in endocrine diseases.[1]

The interrelationship between lipo-health and endocrine function is particularly relevant in the context of the adrenal glands. In this chapter, we delineate the role of adrenal hormones in the regulation of lipid metabolism and describe the lipid alterations seen in disorders of adrenal function.

ADRENAL GLANDS—PHYSIOLOGY

The adrenals are small endocrine glands situated above the kidneys and are composed of the outer adrenal cortex and inner adrenal medulla. The adrenal cortex and medulla have distinct embryological origins and physiological functions. The adrenal cortex is derived from mesoderm while the medulla is of ectodermal origin. The cortex is further composed of three layers involved in the production of steroid hormones and includes:
1. Zona glomerulosa that primarily secretes mineralocorticoid aldosterone
2. Zona fasciculata that secretes glucocorticoids, including cortisol
3. Zona reticularis that secretes adrenal androgens, including dehydroepiandrosterone (DHEA), DHEA sulfate (DHEAS), and androstenedione.

The function of the adrenal cortex is regulated by the hypothalamus and pituitary via adrenocorticotropic hormone (ACTH). On the other hand, the inner medulla secretes catecholamines, adrenaline and noradrenaline, in response to sympathetic nervous system stimulation.

LIPIDS AS A PRECURSOR OF ADRENAL HORMONES

Lipids have diverse physiological functions, including maintaining structural integrity and fluidity of cell membranes and its role in cell signaling, nerve conduction, and intracellular transport. In addition, cholesterol serves as a precursor for hormones, vitamin D, and bile acids.[2]

The adrenal cortex has a distinct yellow color due to its extremely high lipid content.[3] The adrenal cortical cells are specialized in steroid biosynthesis, are rich in mitochondria and smooth endoplasmic reticulum, and contain a high content of intracellular lipid droplets that store cholesteryl esters. They readily take up cholesterol, which serves as the common precursor molecule for adrenal cortical hormones, including glucocorticoids, mineralocorticoids, and adrenal androgens. Flowchart 1 depicts the steroid hormone biosynthetic pathway.

The steroidogenic acute regulatory protein (StAR) mediates the transport of cholesterol into inner mitochondrial membrane where it is utilized for hormone synthesis. Deficiency of the StAR protein results in a rare form of lipoid congenital hyperplasia characterized by severe adrenal insufficiency and significantly enlarged adrenal glands.[4]

EFFECTS OF GLUCOCORTICOIDS ON LIPID METABOLISM

The adrenal steroid hormones, including glucocorticoids, mineralocorticoids, and adrenal androgens regulate lipid and lipoprotein metabolism in several ways. Glucocorticoids play a significant role in energy metabolism and regulate the metabolism of glucose, fat, and protein in conjunction with other hormones such as insulin, glucagon, and thyroid hormones. In fact, it has been shown that glucocorticoids can modulate the expression of almost 10% of human genes.

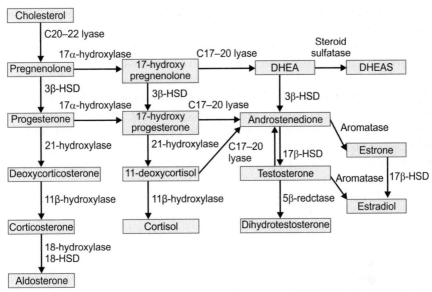

HSD, hydroxysteroid dehydrogenase; DHEA, dehydroepiandrosterone; DHEAS, dehydroepiandrosterone sulfate.

FLOWCHART 1: Steroid biosynthesis pathway.

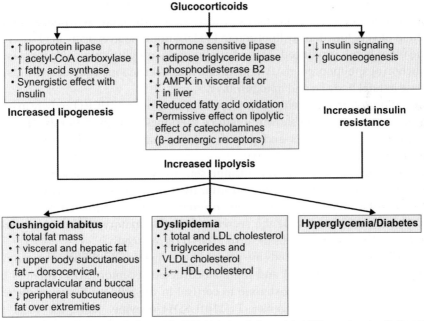

CoA, coenzyme A; LDL, low-density lipoprotein; HDL, high-density lipoprotein; VLDL, very low-density lipoprotein; AMPK, adenosine monophosphate-activated protein kinase.

FLOWCHART 2: Effects of glucocorticoids on adipose tissue and lipid metabolism.

Glucocorticoids regulate adipose tissue distribution and function, and lipid metabolism in several ways and these are depicted in flowchart 2:[5]

- *Increased adipogenesis:* They increase the differentiation of adipocyte precursors and promote fat deposition, especially visceral and abdominal subcutaneous fat. Other fat depots such as dorsocervical, supraclavicular, and buccal fat pads are also sensitive to the adipogenic effect of glucocorticoids
- *Increased lipogenesis:* They increase the expression and activity of intravascular lipoprotein lipase that hydrolyzes the breakdown of triglycerides into fatty acids and glycerol. The resultant increase in adipose tissue uptake of fatty acids and glycerol promotes lipogenesis and increased fat storage in visceral, abdominal, and upper body subcutaneous depots. Glucocorticoids act synergistically with insulin to stimulate acetyl coenzyme A (CoA) carboxylase and fatty acid synthase to further increase lipogenesis[6]
- *Increased lipolysis:* While lipogenesis is increased, glucocorticoids also increase lipolysis by upregulating the activity of hormone sensitive lipase and adipose triglyceride lipase. On the other hand, they inhibit adenosine monophosphate-activated protein kinase (AMPK) and phosphodiesterase 3B that further contribute to their lipolytic effect.[7] They also have a permissive effect on the lipolytic effects of catecholamines, mediated via β-adrenergic receptors, and growth hormone as well.

Therefore, both lipogenesis and lipolysis are increased. Adipogenesis and lipogenesis are predominantly increased in central fat depots; the peripheral adipose tissue is more sensitive to their lipolytic effect.[5] The effect on hepatic lipid metabolism is less well understood. Lipogenesis is increased, with increased production and secretion of very low-density lipoprotein (VLDL) from the liver. Fatty acid oxidation, on the other hand, is reduced. Among apolipoproteins, glucocorticoids increase the production of apolipoprotein AIV and AI. The net effect action of glucocorticoids is an increase in total body fat and lipid turnover.[7]

In addition, glucocorticoids reduce uncoupling protein 1 (UCP1) activity in brown adipocytes and have been shown to reduce thermogenic activity in rats. Thus, they may reduce thermogenesis and promote shift toward white adipocytes, but the significance in humans in not known.

Glucocorticoids also regulate insulin sensitivity and glucose metabolism by decreasing the peripheral uptake and utilization of glucose and increasing gluconeogenesis. The adipose tissue inflammatory activity is also modulated. They increase the expression of leptin while the secretion of inflammatory cytokines interleukin (IL)-6, IL-8, and tumor necrosis factor-α (TNF-α) is reduced.

The effects of glucocorticoids are primarily mediated via the nuclear receptors—glucocorticoid receptor (GR) and mineralocorticoid receptor (MR). There is local conversion of inactive corticosterone to cortisol in the adipose tissue mediated by 11β-hydroxysteroid dehydrogenase-1 (11β-HSD1) enzyme. Since the local concentration of cortisol in adipose tissue is high, it acts via both GR and MR. While GR activation reduces release of proinflammatory adipocytokines, MR activation has the opposite effect. MR activation is now understood to play a significant role in the pathophysiology of obesity, hypertension, and dysmetabolism.[7] Selective agonist of the GR, dexamethasone, and selective antagonists of the MR, eplerenone, reduce secretion of proinflammatory adipokines.

Polymorphisms of the GR are associated with variations in glucocorticoid sensitivity. These have been associated with body mass index (BMI), blood pressure, blood glucose, total and LDL cholesterol, and triglycerides. Glucocorticoid resistance is linked to less visceral obesity, lower fasting insulin, lower cholesterol, and a healthier metabolic profile, while greater responsiveness to glucocorticoids is associated with increased CV risk.[8]

CUSHING'S SYNDROME—LIPID PHENOTYPE

Chronic glucocorticoid excess or Cushing's syndrome can result from exogenous systemic glucocorticoid therapy or endogenous causes, including ACTH secreting tumors (pituitary or ectopic) or cortisol hypersecretion from adrenal lesions. Cushing's syndrome is typically associated with increased central and visceral fat deposition but a depletion of peripheral subcutaneous fat in extremities. The central adiposity is accompanied by increased buccal, dorsocervical and supraclavicular fat, which gives rise to the characteristic Cushingoid features that are considered important clinical clues of hypercortisolism.[5]

In addition to weight gain and central adiposity, chronic glucocorticoid excess is also associated with significant insulin resistance, metabolic syndrome, hyperglycemia or diabetes, hypertension, hypercoagulability, and dyslipidemia. Dyslipidemia results from both the direct effects of hypercortisolism on lipid metabolism as well as due to insulin resistance and diabetes. It also contributes to the development of nonalcoholic fatty liver disease. Both exogenous and endogenous Cushing's syndrome have been associated with increased incidence of hepatic steatosis.

Dyslipidemia is Cushing's Syndrome

Chronic glucocorticoid excess can cause secondary dyslipidemia, but the severity of lipid abnormalities is highly variable in both exogenous and endogenous hypercortisolism.[9] Reports of lipid alterations in Cushing's syndrome vary based on patient characteristics and the severity of disease. Patients with endogenous hypercortisolism have elevated total and LDL cholesterol, elevated triglycerides, and VLDL cholesterol, while the high-density lipoprotein (HDL) levels are not significantly altered.[9] Lipoprotein (a) may also be elevated.

Some of the potential mechanisms contributing to the lipid alterations in hypercortisolism include:

- *Low-density lipoprotein cholesterol:* Glucocorticoids decrease the expression of hepatic LDL receptor and decrease LDL clearance. This may contribute to the increased plasma LDL cholesterol levels[9]
- *Triglycerides:* Glucocorticoids increase hepatic acetyl-CoA carboxylase and fatty acid synthase. Triglyceride synthesis in the liver is increased, apo B degradation is reduced and there is increased formation and secretion of VLDL, while VLDL clearance is unaltered.[6] The increased VLDL production results in increase in both serum triglycerides and LDL cholesterol. Glucocorticoid excess also results in increased adipose tissue lipolysis, with increase in circulating free fatty acids.[10] An increased transport of fatty acids from adipose tissue to liver may also contribute

to increased secretion of VLDL from the liver, but this has not been clearly documented
- *High-density lipoprotein cholesterol*: The synthesis and secretion of apo A1 is increased. In addition, hepatic lipase is inhibited while lecithin–cholesterol acyltransferase (LCAT) is inhibited. This may result in increase in HDL cholesterol.[11] However, significant changes in HDL cholesterol have not been reported.

The total and LDL cholesterol levels seem to correlate with the severity of hypercortisolism and contribute to increase CV risk. While Cushing's syndrome is not associated with low HDL cholesterol, lipid changes in subclinical Cushing's syndrome seem to replicate metabolic syndrome with increased triglycerides and low HDL cholesterol.[12] In individuals with hypopituitarism who were on glucocorticoid replacement, a dose-response relationship was seen between steroid dose and weight, BMI, total and LDL cholesterol, and triglycerides, suggesting that higher doses are associated with greater dyslipidemia. However, in a large survey of 15,004 patients using exogenous glucocorticoids, dyslipidemia was not reported. Exogenous glucocorticoids seem to be associated with dyslipidemia particularly in those individuals who exhibit Cushingoid features.[13]

Insulin resistance and secondary diabetes associated with chronic hypercortisolism further alter the lipid and lipoprotein abnormalities. In addition, Cushing's syndrome may be variably associated with abnormalities in other hormones including growth hormone, prolactin and thyroid hormones, estrogen, or testosterone. These may also modulate lipid parameters.

Cardiovascular Risk in Cushing's Syndrome

Chronic glucocorticoid excess presents a constellation of high CV risk environment with central obesity, insulin resistance, diabetes, hypertension, dyslipidemia, endothelial dysfunction, hypercoagulability, and inflammation. The global CV risk was estimated to be high or very high in almost 80% patients with Cushing's syndrome in a large cohort.[14] Several reports suggest that these patients have higher carotid intima media thickness and coronary artery calcium scores and CV event rates are higher (hazard ratio of 3.7 for myocardial infarction and 2.0 for stroke) and these remain elevated even after treatment of Cushing's syndrome.[12,15] They have a higher mortality rate compared to age and gender-matched controls, largely contributed by CV mortality.[16] The increased risk for atherosclerotic CV disease (ASCVD) and ASCVD-related mortality is multifactorial and is seen even long after achieving remission of hypercortisolism.[17]

Does Treatment of Cushing's Syndrome Improve Dyslipidemia?

Several studies have reported improvements in serum lipids when hypercortisolism is treated, with either medical or surgical management. LDL cholesterol is significantly reduced. However, some reports suggest small to no improvement in lipid profile after achieving remission or cure in Cushing's syndrome. Medical therapies for hypercortisolism such as ketoconazole or mitotane may also impact lipid profile, as discussed in subsequent section. More importantly, the CV risk remains elevated even after achieving remission in Cushing's syndrome patients.[17]

Impact of Medical Therapy for Cushing's Syndrome on Lipid Parameters

Several drugs may be used to reduce cortisol levels in endogenous Cushing's syndrome, including ketoconazole, mitotane, and metyrapone.
- *Ketoconazole:* Ketoconazole blocks several enzymes in cortisol synthesis pathway and reduces serum cortisol levels. In addition, it also blocks cholesterol biosynthesis by inhibiting the conversion of methyl sterols to cholesterol. In fact, ketoconazole was used for lowering of serum lipids in patients with familial hypercholesterolemia before the advent of statins.[18] Use of ketoconazole may lead to improvement in lipid parameters in patients with Cushing's syndrome
- *Mitotane:* On the other hand, mitotane which is used in adrenocortical carcinoma or refractory cases, increases cholesterol levels by reducing the production of oxysterols in liver and increasing the activity of 3-hydroxy-3-methylglutaryl-CoA (HMG-CoA) reductase. Thus, it leads to significant increase in total and LDL cholesterol and apo B, while triglycerides, HDL cholesterol and lipoprotein (a) are not affected.[13]

Management of Dyslipidemia in Cushing's Syndrome

There is a lack of specific studies addressing the management of dyslipidemia in Cushing's syndrome and therefore, there is no clear consensus. It is important to note that CV risk is significantly elevated due to multiple factors and persists even after remission of hypercortisolism. Therefore, good clinical sense suggests that these individuals should be assessed for CV risk and they should be considered for aggressive multifactorial management for CV risk factors.[13] This would include optimization of glycemic control, blood pressure control, and use of lipid-lowering drugs. CV risk assessment can guide the use of lipid-lowering drugs. Statins remain the first-choice hypolipidemic drugs.

Safety Concerns with Statins

- Cushing's syndrome patients often have proximal myopathy and may be more susceptible to statin-induced myopathy. However, this has not been clearly documented
- *Drug interactions with ketoconazole:* Ketoconazole inhibits several hepatic P450 enzymes including *CYP3A4*. Since many statins such as atorvastatin, simvastatin, and lovastatin are metabolized by *CYP3A4*, their plasma concentrations may be elevated with resultant increased risk of myopathy. However, there is no interaction with rosuvastatin or pravastatin that is not metabolized via *CYP3A4*.[13]

ROLE OF GLUCOCORTICOIDS IN OBESITY

There exist several similarities in the phenotype of central obesity and Cushing's syndrome. It is hypothesized that abnormal glucocorticoid physiology may be playing a role in pathophysiology of obesity, leading to the description of visceral obesity as "Cushing's disease of the omentum".[5]

Chronic stress and inflammation are associated with increased activity of the hypothalamic–pituitary–adrenal axis and increased cortisol production and turnover.

However, serum cortisol levels are not increased in obese individuals, though the loss of diurnal variation of serum cortisol is associated with waist hip ratio. Many obese individuals may have inadequately suppressed morning cortisol on overnight dexamethasone suppression test.[5]

In addition, overexpression of 11β-HSD1 that mediates local conversion of cortisone to active cortisol, thus resulting in increased local production of glucocorticoids, has been implicated in obesity, dyslipidemia, and insulin resistance. However, it is unclear if higher 11β-HSD1 activity is a contributing factor to obesity or a compensatory mechanism. Meanwhile, 11β-HSD2 activity also seems to be increased with resultant increase in cortisol turnover. Pharmacological inhibition of 11β-HSD1 may lead to weight loss, improved lipid parameters and increased insulin sensitivity.

LIPID PARAMETERS IN ADRENAL INSUFFICIENCY

Adrenal glucocorticoids are needed for the optimal activity of enzymes that participate in intestinal triglyceride synthesis. Consequently, patients with Addison's disease (adrenocortical inefficiency) may report steatorrhea that improves with steroid replacement. Serum lipid changes have not been documented.

Do Statins Affect Adrenal Function?

Since statins and newer lipid lowering drugs such as proprotein convertase subtilisin/kexin 9 (PCSK9) inhibitors cause significant reductions in cholesterol, a theoretical concern would be their impact on adrenal and gonadal hormogenesis. However, LDL receptor knockout mice do not demonstrate any abnormalities in adrenal or gonadal steroid hormone production.[2] Similarly, most studies with statins or PCSK9 inhibitors do no suggest any adverse effect.[1]

EFFECT OF ADRENAL ANDROGENS ON LIPID PARAMETERS

The role of adrenal androgens in lipid regulation is less clear. The effects of DHEA and DHEAS are mediated via conversion to more potent sex steroids that regulate insulin sensitivity and metabolism. However, studies with DHEA supplementation have failed to report benefits on insulin sensitivity, weight, or lipids; and one study in patients with adrenal insufficiency reported an unfavorable effect on lipids with reduction in HDL cholesterol.[19]

While lipid metabolism may not be affected by congenital adrenal hyperplasia (CAH), most patients are treated with long-term glucocorticoid treatment. Several studies report increased total and LDL cholesterol and triglycerides in CAH patients compared to controls.[20]

EFFECT OF MINERALOCORTICOIDS ON LIPIDS

Aldosterone does not have any direct impact on lipid metabolism, but plays an important role in mediating blood pressure control, endothelial function, insulin sensitivity, and chronic inflammation. Both mineralocorticoids and glucocorticoids act via the MR to increase adipogenesis and inflammatory activity. Primary hyperaldosteronism is associated with hypertension, insulin resistance, and increased CV risk but consistent changes in lipids have not been reported.[21]

ADRENAL MEDULLA—EFFECT ON LIPID METABOLISM

Catecholamines increase thermogenesis in brown adipose tissue via β2-adrenergic receptors and may induce browning of white adipocytes. Agonists of the β2-adrenergic receptors are currently being explored for their role in obesity.

Catecholamines, epinephrine and norepinephrine have a predominant lipolytic effect, by increasing cyclic AMP levels and activity of hormone-sensitive lipase. In addition, they inhibit insulin secretion and decrease insulin sensitivity, which further increases lipolysis. Catecholamine-secreting tumors or pheochromocytomas may be associated with lower body fat, carbohydrate intolerance, elevated free fatty acids, and lower HDL cholesterol, but changes in LDL cholesterol or triglycerides have not been reported. The carbohydrate tolerance and free fatty acid levels return to normal after surgical resection of the tumor.[22]

LIPID CONTENT OF ADRENALS—IMAGING OF ADRENAL TUMORS

Adrenal lesions include adenomas, adrenocortical carcinomas, pheochromocytomas, metastasis, myelolipomas, lymphomas, cysts or pseudocysts, hemorrhage, infections, or nodular hyperplasia. The primary concern on imaging is to distinguish benign adenomas from malignant lesions. Most adrenal adenomas have intracytoplasmic fat, which differentiates them from malignant or metastatic lesions.[23] These can be easily identified in nonenhanced computed tomography (CT) and magnetic resonance imaging (MRI).

On noncontrast CT, most adenomas have a low attenuation, below 10 HU (Hounsfield unit) due to their fat content. But 10–40% adenomas have a higher attenuation and therefore, noncontrast CT may be indeterminate. Contrast-enhanced images may assist as adenomas have significant arterial enhancement and rapid washout of contrast. However, some pheochromocytomas and metastatic lesions have similar characteristics.[24]

Fat can be depicted in routine fat-suppressed MRI that can detect macroscopic fat. However, it may not pick up microscopic intracellular fat that can be demonstrated via the use of chemical shift MRI. The precession frequencies of water and lipid molecules are different and can be easily distinguished during the acquisition sequence of chemical shift MRI. Intracellular fat is detected as a signal drop on opposed-phase images with a darker appearance compared to in-phase images and the microscopic fat content can also be quantified.[23] Therefore, adenomas have a signal drop on chemical shift MRI, which has a high sensitivity and specificity in differentiating them from malignancies or other lesions which are lipid-poor.

Certain adrenal tumors, adrenal myelolipomas, have significant macroscopic fat and are very easily diagnosed on imaging. They appear as lesions with significant fat attenuation on CT and loss of signal on fat-saturated MRI. The differential diagnosis of such lesions includes lipomas, liposarcomas, and pheochromocytomas that have undergone significant fat degeneration.[24]

CONCLUSION

Glucocorticoids are key regulators of energy metabolism and affect lipid and lipoprotein metabolism through several mechanisms. Cushing's syndrome is associated with increased visceral and upper body fat, increased lipogenesis as well as increased lipolysis. The resultant changes in serum lipids include increase in total and LDL cholesterol and triglycerides. In addition, patients with chronic glucocorticoid excess also have abnormal glucose metabolism, central obesity, hypertension, hypercoagulability, and endothelial dysfunction. Cardiovascular risk and mortality are significantly elevated, even after remission of hypercortisolism. This calls for aggressive multifactorial risk factor management with therapy targeted at optimization of glycemic control, blood pressure and lipids, and lifestyle modification, in addition to management of Cushing's syndrome.

REFERENCES

1. Kalra S, Priya G. Lipocrinology—the relationship between lipids and endocrine function. Drugs Context. 2018;7:212514.
2. Berg JM, Tymoczko JL, Stryer L. Section 26.4, Important Derivatives of Cholesterol Include Bile Salts and Steroid Hormones. In: Berg JM, Tymoczko JL, Stryer L (Eds). Biochemistry, 5th edition. New York: W H Freeman; 2002.
3. Blaschko H, Firemark H, Smith AD, et al. Lipids of the adrenal medulla: Lysolecithin, a characteristic constituent of chromaffin granules. Biochem J. 1967;104(2):545-9.
4. Kim CJ. Congenital lipoid adrenal hyperplasia. Ann Pediatr Endocrinol Metab. 2014;19(4):179-83.
5. Lee MJ, Pramyothin P, Karastergiou K, et al. Deconstructing the roles of glucocorticoids in adipose tissue biology and the development of central obesity. Biochim Biophys Acta. 2014;1842(3):473-81.
6. de Guia RM, Herzig S. How Do Glucocorticoids Regulate Lipid Metabolism? Adv Exp Med Biol. 2015;872:127-44.
7. Macfarlane DP, Forbes S, Walker BR. Glucocorticoids and fatty acid metabolism in humans: fuelling fat redistribution in the metabolic syndrome. J Endocrinol. 2008;197(2):189-204.
8. Yan YX, Dong J, Wu LJ, et al. Associations between polymorphisms in the glucocorticoid-receptor gene and cardiovascular risk factors in a Chinese population. J Epidemiol. 2013;23(5):389-95.
9. Gälman C, Angelin B, Rudling M. Prolonged stimulation of the adrenals by corticotropin suppresses hepatic low-density lipoprotein and high-density lipoprotein receptors and increases plasma cholesterol. Endocrinology. 2002;143(5):1809-16.
10. Peckett AJ, Wright DC, Riddell MC. The effects of glucocorticoids on adipose tissue lipid metabolism. Metabolism. 2011;60(11):1500-10.
11. Feingold K, Brinton EA, Grunfeld C. The effect of endocrine disorders on lipids and lipoproteins. In: De Groot LJ, Chrousos G, Dungan K, et al. (Eds). Endotext [Internet]. South Dartmouth (MA): MDText.com, Inc.; 2000-2017.
12. Arnaldi G, Scandali VM, Trementino L, et al. Pathophysiology of dyslipidemia in Cushing's syndrome. Neuroendocrinology. 2010;92 Suppl 1:86-90.
13. Greenman Y. Management of dyslipidemia in Cushing's syndrome. Neuroendocrinology. 2010;92 Suppl 1:91-5.
14. Mancini T, Kola B, Mantero F, et al. High cardiovascular risk in patients with Cushing's syndrome according to 1999 WHO/ISH guidelines. Clin Endocrinol. 2004;61:768-77.
15. Barahona MJ, Resmini E, Viladés D, et al. Coronary artery disease detected by multislice computed tomography in patients after long-term cure of Cushing's syndrome. J Clin Endocrinol Metab. 2013;98(3):1093-9.
16. Ntali G, Asimakopoulou A, Siamatras T, et al. Mortality in Cushing's syndrome: systematic analysis of a large series with prolonged follow-up. Eur J Endocrinol. 2013;169(5):715-23.

17. Clayton RN, Jones PW, Reulen RC, et al. Mortality in patients with Cushing's disease more than 10 years after remission: a multicentre, multinational, retrospective cohort study. Lancet Diabetes Endocrinol. 2016;4(7):569-76.
18. Gylling H, Vanhanen H, Miettinen TA. Hypolipidemic effect and mechanism of ketoconazole without and with cholestyramine in familial hypercholesterolemia. Metabolism. 1991;40(1):35-41.
19. Srinivasan M, Irving BA, Dhatariya K, et al. Effect of dehydroepiandrosterone replacement on lipoprotein profile in hypoadrenal women. J Clin Endocrinol Metab. 2009;94(3):761-4.
20. Botero D, Arango A, Danon M, et al. Lipid profile in congenital adrenal hyperplasia. Metabolism. 2000;49(6):790-3.
21. Pimenta E, Calhoun DA. Aldosterone and metabolic dysfunction: an unresolved issue. Hypertension. 2009;53(4):585-6.
22. Okamura T, Nakajima Y, Satoh T, et al. Changes in visceral and subcutaneous fat mass in patients with pheochromocytoma. Metabolism. 2015;64(6):706-12.
23. Adam SZ, Nikolaidis P, Horowitz JM, et al. Chemical Shift MR Imaging of the Adrenal Gland: Principles, Pitfalls, and Applications. Radiographics. 2016;36(2):414-32.
24. Herr K, Muglia VF, Koff WJ, et al. Imaging of the adrenal gland lesions. Radiologia Brasileira. 2014;47(4):228-39.

Lipo-health and the Endocrine System: Reproductive System

KVS Hari Kumar

ABSTRACT

Reproductive system and lipids have close relationship in the physiology of all living organisms. The studies looking from the evolutionary perspective have described these links even in nematodes, insects, and other mammals. The lipid health (lipo-health) determines the fertility potential and also the life span in many living species. Lipids have higher energy content in comparison to proteins and carbohydrates. The process of reproduction is an energy-intensive process, which is supported by the energy derived from the lipids. Cholesterol is the precursor for all steroidogenic hormones involved in the development and functioning of the reproductive organs. Aging affects lipid metabolism and reproductive capacity either directly or indirectly through obesity and other metabolic disorders. The deficiency of gonadal hormones affects the lipo-health of an individual. In this chapter, we discuss the interactions between the reproductive system and lipid health along with the observed changes in various pathophysiological states.

INTRODUCTION

Lipids and reproductive system share a bidirectional relationship with close interaction between each other in their physiology. Lipids have an important role in the physiology and the normal functioning of the reproductive system. All gonadal hormones are derivatives of cholesterol and are synthesized in gonads and adrenal glands. Numerous studies have shown that inadequate secretion of gonadal hormones results in obesity and increased fat mass. This was once considered as an essential mechanism that contributed toward increased longevity-associated with hypogonadism. However, an inverse situation is observed with the development of obesity and insulin resistance due to the deposition of excess fat tissue in hypogonadal states. The mediators and hormonal links between the reproductive system, lipids, and aging have been poorly understood. The evolutionary link connecting reproductive and lipid systems is an important trade-off between somatic maintenance, reproduction, survival, and fat stores. A close understanding of these interactions could help in solving many mysteries pertaining to metabolic disorders.

EVOLUTIONARY PERSPECTIVE

The observational studies and the evolutionary history of living organisms suggest that life span is intricately linked to reproduction and lipid stores.[1] Species with curtailed reproduction survive longer than those with higher reproductive effort. Previous studies involving mammals demonstrated that gonadectomy results in obesity, increased fat mass, and a longer life span. A similar finding has been observed even in insects and lower mammals like rats, cats, and monkeys. The signals due to hypogonadism not only affect the adipose tissue but also the aging processes. Steroid hormones are the possible mediators of this physiological adaptive mechanism. The molecular connections between life span and reproduction are mediated by insulin-like growth factor 1 (IGF-1) and steroid signaling pathways. Forkhead box O (FOXO) and phosphatase and tensin homolog (PTEN) proteins are components of IGF-1 signaling system that play a significant role in this pathway. Enhanced fat storage in response to life span promoting mutations is necessary for somatic maintenance. However, excess of fat beyond a critical threshold leads to the risk of obesity, cancer, diabetes, and cardiovascular disorders. Thus, it is unclear from the evolutionary perspective, whether the links between these processes are casual or causal in their nature.

PHYSIOLOGICAL LINKS

Lipids are hydrophobic molecules and have diverse biological roles including being an important cellular energy source. They are also important constituents in the anchorage of cell membranes and play a pivotal role in intracellular cell signaling. The traditional role of lipids is to maintain the reproduction and not divert themselves to somatic growth and other menial tasks.

Adipose tissue and reproductive organs are in close synchrony at several levels. While lipids and adipose tissue play a vital role in gonadal organ development and function, hormone synthesis and metabolism, gonadal hormones, in turn, regulate lipid physiology in multiple ways. These bidirectional physiological links are described in subsequent sections.

Role of Lipids in Reproductive Physiology

Lipids play a vital role in several aspects of reproductive physiology, including, steroid hormonogenesis, spermatogenesis and sperm maturation, oogenesis and oocyte maturation, and fertilization as depicted in flowchart 1. Cholesterol is the precursor for the synthesis of gonadal steroids, glucocorticoids, and mineralocorticoids in the adrenals and gonads and is derived by the hormone producing cells from circulation or synthesized de novo. The transport of cholesterol from outer to inner mitochondrial membrane is regulated by the steroidogenic acute regulatory (StAR) protein. Additionally, the development of the reproductive organs is dependent on an adequate concentration of local and systemic sex hormones.

SECTION 1: Lipids in Endocrinology

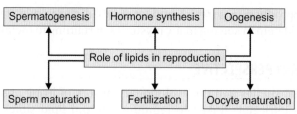

FLOWCHART 1: Lipids in reproduction.

TABLE 1 Physiological actions of reproductive hormones on lipids

Hormone	Mechanism	Effect
Testosterone	• Upregulates SRB-1 and hepatic lipase • Downregulates LDL receptors • Inhibits lipid uptake • Stimulate lipolysis • Decreases lipogenesis	• Reduced HDL-C • Increased LDL-C
Estrogen	• Upregulates LDL receptor expression • Inhibits PCSK9 • Inhibits hepatic lipase • Stimulates Apo-A1	• Reduces LDL • Increases HDL especially HDL2
Progesterone	• Induces hepatic lipase	• Reduced HDL
DHEA	• Precursor of estrogen and testosterone	• Increased HDL, Apo-A1 • Decreased total cholesterol

apoA-I, apolipoprotein A-I; DHEA, dehydroepiandrosterone; HDL, high-density lipoprotein; LDL, low-density lipoprotein; PCSK9, proprotein convertase subtilisin/kexin type-9; SRB-1, scavenger receptor B-1

Effects of Gonadal Hormones on Lipid Metabolism

Testosterone and estrogen are the two predominant gonadal hormones in males and females, respectively. Other hormones secreted from the gonads include progesterone and dehydroepiandrosterone (DHEA). Testosterone upregulates hepatic lipase and scavenger receptor B-1 (SRB-1) which are involved in the catabolism of high-density lipoprotein cholesterol (HDL-C) thereby, reducing the level of HDL-C. Testosterone also counters the estrogen-mediated low-density lipoprotein (LDL) receptor upregulation, resulting in increased LDL-C. Estrogen has beneficial effects on the lipids and is responsible for the cardiovascular protection in menstruating females. Estrogen increases HDL-C levels by stimulating the synthesis of Apo-A1 and inhibiting the expression of SRB-1 and hepatic lipase. Estrogen reduces the LDL-C levels by multiple mechanisms including upregulation and reduced degradation of LDL receptors and inhibition of proprotein convertase subtilisin/kexin type-9 (PCSK-9) enzyme. The effect of progestogenic compounds on lipids is mediated through their binding on to the androgen receptor and may be variable. DHEA has a minimal direct effect on the lipid metabolism and its effects are mediated primarily via conversion to more potent androgens. Table 1 summarizes lipid effects of various reproductive hormones.

LIPO-HEALTH DURING PHASES OF REPRODUCTIVE LIFE

The reproductive system functions at different tempos during various stages in the life span of an individual. These include a dormant phase prior to puberty, hyperactive stage during adulthood, and a stage of declining function in the elderly. The lipid health parallels these changes in the reproductive system and these lipid alterations are described in subsequent sections.

Gonadal Development

The fertilization of the ovum and subsequent development of embryo into fetus is an energy-intensive process. The energy for this is derived from the intracellular lipids stored in the oocyte. Fatty acids generated by lipolysis are metabolized in the mitochondria for adenosine triphosphate (ATP) production.[2] The fatty acid milieu in the cumulus–oocyte complex is important for the developmental competence of the oocyte and embryo. The developing gonad produces several hormones that mediate sexual differentiation resulting in the phenotypic sex of the fetus. The local production of testosterone in males is essential for the differentiation of Wolffian structures while dihydrotestosterone determines androgenization of external genitalia. It follows that disorders leading to inadequate testosterone production in utero are associated with disorders of sexual differentiation (DSD) in male fetuses. On the other hand, the gonadal differentiation in females is mostly a passive process and the ovaries are generally quiescent till puberty. Likewise, excess androgen exposure of female fetus can lead to DSD.

Puberty

Puberty is a process of sexual maturation and preparation of the gonadal and genital system for future reproduction. There is a secular trend of early puberty observed in the last couple of decades coinciding with the epidemic of obesity. It is important to reach a critical body weight or body fat percentage for the activation of the hypothalamo-pituitary-gonadal pulse generator. Leptin hormone produced from adipocytes shows gradual peaking prior to the onset of puberty establishing a definite link between the adipocytes and puberty. During the process of puberty, girls and boys undergo significant changes in the distribution of adipose tissue and plasma lipid levels. The quantum of adipose tissue acquisition during puberty might influence the future cardiovascular risk in children. Fat free mass accounts for the major portion of weight gain during puberty in comparison to fat mass. As far as adipose tissue mass is concerned, the central or visceral fat is not increased while a minor increase is observed in the subcutaneous adipose tissue. Lipid profile changes observed during different stages of puberty are influenced by the race and sex of the child. In general, there is a decrease in the levels of total cholesterol, LDL-C, and non-HDL cholesterol in both males and females.[3] HDL-C and triglycerides (TG) are not changed in females, whereas the former is reduced and the latter is increased in males. Females and non-black youth have higher lipid levels than their counterparts, respectively. It is important to identify the pubertal stage at the time of assessment of lipid profile in children.

Adults

Adipocytes, whether located in the visceral and subcutaneous tissue, have androgen and estrogen receptors mediating their respective actions. The lipo-health of an individual during adult life is influenced by lifestyle, obesity, and other metabolic disorders. The same has been described in detail in other chapters of the book. As a broad principle, estrogens result in antiatherogenic lipid profile, whereas androgens result in proatherogenic changes. The high estrogen levels offer some protection to adult menstruating females from cardiovascular disorders.

Aging

Aging induces many abnormalities in the physiology of lipids and the reproductive system. Aging is associated with obesity, hypogonadism, and increased visceral adipose tissue in both males and females. There is a bidirectional link between the declining gonadal functions seen with aging and obesity with many intermediary mechanisms. The observed lipid changes are mediated either directly by aging or indirectly by associated obesity and hypogonadism. The detailed interactions between the cessation of gonadal function and lipid health are described subsequently.

GONADOPAUSE AND LIPO-HEALTH

The cessation of reproductive function is a definite event in females and a gradual event in the males. Menopause occurs at approximately 50 years of age and there is a rapid decline in the production of female sex hormones. Male climacteric is a gradual process with a declining testosterone level at a rate of 5–10% per annum from fifth decade onward. The resulting hypogonadism affects the lipo-health of an individual leading to increased propensity to metabolic and cardiovascular disorders.

Menopause

The menopausal transition (MT) leads to a drastic decline in estradiol levels coupled with a relative rise in the level of androgens. There is an increase in fat mass, particularly visceral fat, and reduction in skeletal mass in postmenopausal females.[4] Visceral fat has higher rates of lipolysis and is associated with increased flux of free fatty acids to the liver which promotes insulin resistance. Molecular studies have also demonstrated differences in the metabolism of pre- and postmenopausal adipocytes. These include the expression of genes influencing insulin sensitivity, peroxisome proliferator-activated receptor, circadian rhythms, and fatty acid transporter genes. MT is also associated with increased risk of obesity and diabetes mellitus, which may further increase the risk of dyslipidemia. Recent studies have demonstrated that the dyslipidemia in menopausal females is independent of confounding factors such as age, body mass index, obesity, glycemia, smoking, alcohol, and reduced physical activity. In MT, there may be a mild change in total HDL-C, but there is an increase in the subfraction 3 (HDL3) and decrease in subfraction 2 (HDL2). HDL2 is more active in the reverse cholesterol transport when compared with HDL3. Hepatic lipase converts

HDL3 into HDL2 and the activity of this enzyme increases in postmenopausal women as estrogens inhibit this enzyme.

Many observational studies have demonstrated that estrogen replacement therapy (ERT) confers cardiovascular protection in postmenopausal women. However, randomized controlled trials did not replicate this benefit, leading to a concept known as the estrogen paradox. ERT in the immediate postmenopausal phase decreases cardiovascular risk, whereas ERT in late menopausal stage (beyond 10 years) increases cardiovascular risk. Currently, ERT is only recommended for the amelioration of menopausal symptoms and not for cardiovascular protection.

Andropause

The age-related decline in testosterone is contributed by the declining function of Leydig cells and hypothalamo-pituitary-gonadal axis. Typically, these patients have high LDL-C and TG and low HDL-C. Most of these lipid abnormalities revert to normal with sex hormone replacement.[5] Suraphysiological doses of testosterone, however, lead to worsening of the lipid abnormalities as observed in certain athletes with testosterone abuse.

Patients with metabolic syndrome and/or type 2 diabetes may have hypogonadism and low testosterone level. The disease often manifests as erectile dysfunction (ED) and ED is considered a sensitive marker of the endothelial health of the individual. Reduced levels of testosterone result in decreased lipogenesis, increased lipolysis, and reduced lipid uptake. The effect is mediated through lipoprotein lipase, the key enzyme that increases the fatty acid uptake. Testosterone supplementation has resulted in the improvement in the waist circumference and lipids in many patients with late onset hypogonadism. Testosterone replacement also results in the improvement of associated inflammatory markers. Studies have shown that there is an inverse correlation between the testosterone levels and the amount of the visceral adipose tissue.

LIPO-HEALTH IN REPRODUCTIVE DISORDERS

Sex of an individual has multiple facets including gonadal, chromosomal, and psychological sex. Androgens and estrogens influence the psychosexual development of the individual from very early in life. The effect of hypogonadism on lipid health in both men and women has been discussed in the previous section pertaining to gonadopause. The lipid abnormalities observed in certain other reproductive disorders are described below and in table 2.

Precocious Puberty

Early menarche is associated with increased risk of cardiovascular disease in the adulthood. Girls with precocious puberty have higher levels of IGF-1 and insulin which may contribute to insulin resistance and risk of cardiovascular disease. The lipid abnormalities described in these children are typical to that of metabolic syndrome, viz. low HDL-C and high TG.

SECTION 1: Lipids in Endocrinology

TABLE 2 Reproductive disorders and lipid abnormalities

Disorder	Lipid alteration	Effect
Hypogonadism	• Increased LPL activity	• High LDL-C, TG • Low HDL-C
Andropause	• Downregulates LDL receptor expression • Hepatic lipase and SRB-1 decreases	• High LDL-C, TG • Low HDL-C
Menopause	• Increased activity of hepatic lipase and lipoprotein lipase	• Increased TG, VLDL • Increased small, dense LDL • Increased HDL3 and reduced HDL2 • Increased Apo-B
Precocious puberty	• Same as insulin resistance	• Decreased LDL • Increased TG
PCOS	• Hepatic secretion of VLDL • Apo-A1 clearance is increased	• Increased LDL, VLDL, TG, FFA • Decreased HDL, Apo-A1 • Increased small, dense, oxidized LDL

LPL, lipoprotein lipase; LDL, low-density lipoprotein; HDL, high-density lipoprotein; TG, triglycerides; VLDL, very low-density lipoprotein; FFA, free fatty acids; Apo, apolipoprotein; PCOS, polycystic ovary syndrome; SRB-1, scavenger receptor B-1

Polycystic Ovarian Syndrome

Polycystic ovarian syndrome (PCOS) is a common disorder in adolescent and young females that has many long-term cardiovascular and metabolic consequences. A high prevalence of lipid abnormalities has been reported in women with PCOS. These include increased LDL-C, VLDL-cholesterol and TG, and decreased HDL-C.[6] The atherogenicity increases further due to a preponderance of oxidized, small, dense LDL cholesterol particles in the circulation. Lipoprotein (a) and apo-B are also elevated in patients with PCOS. Insulin resistance is the key determinant of all metabolic and lipid abnormalities in patients with PCOS. The contribution of hyperandrogenism to dyslipidemia is controversial with few studies supporting and few others negating this association. Dietary modification, life style measures, and lipid-lowering drugs may be required in PCOS patients for dyslipidemia management.

Sex Chromosomal Disorders

Sex chromosomal disorders include conditions that are affected by the loss, damage or addition of the sex chromosomes, leading to low to absent gonadal function. Turner's syndrome (45,XO) and Klinefelter's syndrome (47,XXY) are the common sex chromosomal disorders in clinical practice. Turner's syndrome is associated with insulin resistance and increased incidence of cardiovascular risk factors. Elevation in total cholesterol has been described and the same is partially ameliorated with the start of ERT.[7] Hypogonadism is the hallmark of the Klinefelter's syndrome and the lipid abnormalities mimic those seen in patients with hypogonadism.[8] The findings include elevated TG and low HDL with no effect on the total cholesterol and LDL cholesterol levels.

Transsexual Disorders

Hormonal therapy is the cornerstone in patients with gender dysphoria and sex reversal surgery. Testosterone and estrogenic preparations are used in female to male (FTM) and male to female (MTF) transsexuals, respectively. In both MTF and FTM patients, there is a long-term use of sex hormones to maintain the appropriate body habitus. The lipid abnormalities observed in transsexuals have not been studied in detail due to few numbers of patients available on long-term hormonal therapy. However, some published case series suggest that the results have been similar to that described in other individuals with the hormone replacement therapy.

CONCLUSION

To conclude, lipids play an important role in the development and functioning of the reproductive system. The multifactorial role includes right from providing energy to the oocyte till late in the adulthood. Cholesterol is the building block for the synthesis of all the vital hormones in the body. The alterations in the lipid metabolism result in the increased risk of atherosclerotic cardiovascular disorders and early identification helps in mitigating the associated risk of morbidity and mortality.

REFERENCES

1. Hansen M, Flatt T, Aguilaniu H. Reproduction, fat metabolism, and life span: what is the connection? Cell Metab. 2013;17(1):10-9.
2. Dunning KR, Russell DL, Robker RL. Lipids and oocyte developmental competence: the role of fatty acids and β-oxidation. Reproduction. 2014;148(1):R15-27.
3. Eissa MA, Mihalopoulos NL, Holubkov R, et al. Changes in fasting lipids during puberty. J Pediatr. 2016;170:199-205.
4. Stefanska A, Bergmann K, Sypniewska G. Metabolic syndrome and menopause: pathophysiology, clinical and diagnostic significance. Adv Clin Chem. 2015;72:1-75.
5. Samaras N, Samaras D, Lang PO, et al. A view of geriatrics through hormones. What is the relation between andropause and well-known geriatric syndromes? Maturitas. 2013;74(3):213-9.
6. Wild RA, Rizzo M, Clifton S, et al. Lipid levels in polycystic ovary syndrome: systematic review and meta-analysis. Fertil Steril. 2011;95(3):1073-9.e1-11.
7. Ross JL, Feuillan P, Long LM, et al. Lipid abnormalities in Turner syndrome. J Pediatr. 1995;126(2):242-5.
8. Lee HS, Park CW, Lee JS, et al. Hypogonadism makes dyslipidemia in Klinefelter's syndrome. J Korean Med Sci. 2017;32(11):1848-51.

CHAPTER 5

Lipo-health and the Endocrine System: Pancreas

Arjin P Jacoby, Jubbin J Jacob

ABSTRACT

Exocrine pancreas secretes several enzymes that are involved in the digestion of dietary lipids. Deficiency of exocrine pancreas, as seen in chronic pancreatitis, is often associated with fat malabsorption and deficiency of fat-soluble vitamins. Pancreatic enzyme replacement therapy ameliorates the resultant malabsorption along with nutrient supplementation. In addition, these patients may also develop secondary diabetes due to islet cell dysfunction. Likewise, disorders of lipid metabolism can affect exocrine pancreatic health. Severe hypertriglyceridemia is known to induce acute pancreatitis and this entity should be considered in the differential diagnosis of patients presenting with acute pancreatitis. The endocrine pancreas is a key regulator of lipid metabolism, with its key hormones, i.e., insulin and glucagon, regulating several enzymes involved in lipogenesis, lipolysis, and fatty acid oxidation. While insulin promotes lipogenesis and reduces lipolysis, the effects of glucagon are generally the opposite. Lipotoxicity has been implicated in insulin resistance and the progressive decline of β-cell function in the pathogenesis of type 2 diabetes mellitus. Amelioration of lipotoxicity and glucotoxicity may be an important strategy to retard the relentless progression of diabetes. Lastly, the lipid effects of glucagon are only beginning to be understood and further work is needed to elucidate its effects as a hypolipidemic agent.

INTRODUCTION

The pancreas, a gland with both endocrine and exocrine functions lies in the inferior aspect of the stomach in the bend of the duodenum. The denser endocrine pancreas, also known as the islets of Langerhans, makes up for just 2% of the whole of the pancreas by volume. The principal hormones secreted by various islet cells clusters include insulin, glucagon, somatostatin, ghrelin and pancreatic polypeptide (PP). The endocrine pancreases are principally concerned with glucose metabolism with insulin and glucagon being the two key players. In addition, these hormones regulate lipid and protein metabolism and work in synchrony with the liver and adipose tissue to maintain metabolic homeostasis.

The pancreas also has an exocrine component, which is primarily concerned with lipid absorption. The role of pancreas in elevating serum lipid levels was first demonstrated in the 1940s by Professor Laurence M Montgomery and colleagues in elegant experiments conducted on depancreatized dogs at the University of California. They found that depancreatized dogs, which are kept alive on insulin, had low lipid levels in the blood. When these dogs were subsequently fed raw pancreas every day, there was an increase in the lipid levels in the blood. Moreover, when they were supplemented with pancreatic juices, it resulted in normalization of lipid levels. These experiments for the first time revealed the importance of pancreatic exocrine secretion in the absorption of lipids from the intestine.[1]

In this chapter, the authors have discussed the physiological role of exocrine pancreas in lipid absorption and described the lipid abnormalities that accompany exocrine pancreatic diseases. Furthermore, the authors provide an overview of the effect of endocrine pancreatic hormones, insulin and glucagon, on lipid metabolism in both health and disease. Abnormal lipid metabolism affects the health of pancreatic β- and α-cells and this has been dealt with in the final part of this chapter.

LIPOCRINOLOGY AND THE EXOCRINE PANCREAS

The exocrine pancreas consists of two cell groups—the acinar cells and the ductal cells, which collectively secrete the pancreatic fluid.[2] The acinar cells principally secrete isotonic saline and acidic digestive enzymes. The ductal cells that comprise of only 5% of the exocrine pancreas, secrete a much larger proportion of the pancreatic fluid. This consists predominantly of alkaline fluids that aim to neutralize the hydrogen ion (H^+)-rich acinar fluid and gastric secretions providing an optimal milieu for effective digestion.[2] Among the various ductal cell groups, the pancreatic ductal epithelial cells play a pivotal role in this neutralization process and its dysfunction has been implicated in several disease processes like acute pancreatitis, chronic pancreatitis and T2DM.[3]

Under physiological conditions following a meal, the exocrine pancreas secretes 1.5 L of an aqueous solution, which contains three groups of enzymes—lipases, amylases, and proteases, involved in the digestion of fat, carbohydrates, and proteins, respectively. In addition to the pancreatic lipases, lipases are secreted in the saliva and stomach. All three together are responsible for fat digestion wherein fat molecules are hydrolyzed and then emulsified with bile acids into micelles and absorbed in the jejunum. Unlike proteins and carbohydrates where extra pancreatic enzyme secretion (salivary and gastric) can compensate for a deficiency of pancreatic enzyme secretion, lipid digestion is significantly impaired in the presence of exocrine pancreatic insufficiency (EPI).[4]

HYPERTRIGLYCERIDEMIA AND ACUTE PANCREATITIS

Hypertriglyceridemia (HTG) is a commonly encountered lipid abnormality frequently associated with other lipid and metabolic derangements. It refers to abnormal fasting plasma triglyceride (TG) measurement that is increased above the 95th percentile for age and sex, with or without any additional quantitative or qualitative lipoprotein abnormalities.[5]

The two main sources of plasma TGs (also known as triacylglycerol) are *exogenous* (i.e., from dietary fat) and carried in chylomicrons, and *endogenous* (from the liver) and carried in very low-density lipoprotein (VLDL) particles. The increase in plasma of TG-rich lipoproteins results from either an increased production from the liver and intestine (by means of up-regulated synthetic and secretory pathways) or through decreased peripheral catabolism (mainly from reduced lipoprotein lipase activity).[6]

The relationship between HTG and the pancreas has been studied extensively. Patients with moderate-to-severe HTG (TG levels >500 mg/dL) are predisposed to acute pancreatitis while patients with acute pancreatitis may have mild to moderate elevations of TG levels. Cameron et al. found lactescent serum in 21% patients with acute pancreatitis. These patients had TG levels ranging from 493 to 7,520 mg/dL.[7] Although the exact pathogenesis is not known, it is thought that the extravascular chylomicrons in the pancreas cause the release of free fatty acids (FFAs), which triggers the inflammation cascade. It is very likely that the FFAs produced within the acinar cells induce mitochondrial toxicity leading to a decrease in acinar ATP (adenosine triphosphate) levels and result in tissue necrosis induced by inhibition of mitochondrial complexes by the FFAs.[8] Hemorrhagic pancreatitis is the most serious, life-threatening complication of severe HTG, particularly if it occurs during pregnancy.[8]

Another common scenario for acute hyperlipidemic pancreatitis is in the setting of poorly controlled diabetes. In type 1 diabetes mellitus (T1DM), the lack of insulin results in a reduced synthesis and activity of the lipoprotein lipase. Meanwhile, in an obese patient with T2DM, there exists a state of insulin resistance which results in reduced clearing of plasma TGs despite apparent abundance in insulin levels.[9] Therefore, acute and severe hyperglycemia may result in TG elevations significant enough to precipitate acute pancreatitis.

Lipid assessment should be routinely done in all patients presenting with acute pancreatitis and it may not be feasible to perform a fasting lipid profile. In fact, TG levels should be assessed at admission as they may subsequently reduce with fasting. Table 1 enlists the features that would increase the clinical suspicion for HTG-induced pancreatitis. When TG levels are very high, pancreatic enzyme levels and blood glucose concentrations may be spuriously low due to interference from lipemic serum.

Initial management of HTG-related pancreatitis is standard with limiting oral intake, pain relief, and aggressive fluid management. In selected patients with severe pancreatitis, who require prolonged fasting, nasojejunal enteral feeding or total parenteral nutrition (TPN), may be initiated.[8] Lipid preparations should be avoided for TPN.

Insulin infusions have often been used in the acute setting cases of HTG-induced pancreatitis. Insulin should be administered along with glucose to avoid hypoglycemia. Insulin acts by increasing lipoprotein lipase activity and rapidly reduces serum TG levels. Insulin infusion is particularly useful in patients with poorly controlled diabetes and HTG. Heparin has also been used in the past for acutely reducing serum TG levels as it increases lipoprotein lipase activity, but the effect is transient. In severe cases, plasmapheresis may be required as it rapidly removes TGs by clearing VLDL and chylomicron particles from the bloodstream. However,

CHAPTER 5: Lipo-health and the Endocrine System: Pancreas

TABLE 1 Clinical features that raise suspicion of hypertriglyceridemia-induced acute pancreatitis

	Factors
Patient history	• History of poorly controlled diabetes • Significant alcohol intake • High carbohydrate intake • Medications predisposing to hypertriglyceridemia (glucocorticoids, isotretinoin, protease inhibitors, tamoxifen, estrogen, propofol, valproic acid) • History of familial combined hyperlipidemia, familial hypertriglyceridemia or familial chylomicronemia, familial dysbetalipoproteinemia • Pregnancy (especially third trimester) • Premature cardiovascular disease
Physical examination	• Lactescent or lipemic serum • Eruptive xanthomas • Lipemia retinalis • Hepatosplenomegaly
Laboratory/ radiological evaluation	• Absence of gallstone disease • Moderate to severe hypertriglyceridemia (>500 mg/dL)*

*Mild-to-moderate hypertriglyceridemia may occur due to the metabolic derangements in acute pancreatitis.

TABLE 2 Management of hypertriglyceridemia-induced acute pancreatitis

Acute	Supportive care	• Limit oral intake • Intravenous hydration • Nasojejunal feeding • Total parenteral nutrition (avoid lipid preparations) • Pain relief
	Target hyper-triglyceridemia	• Insulin infusion (with glucose) • Heparin • Plasmapheresis
Long-term care and prevention	Nonpharmacological	• Lifestyle modification • Avoid alcohol intake • Optimal glycemic control • Avoid drugs causing hypertriglyceridemia • Medium chain triglycerides
	Pharmacological (target hyper-triglyceridemia)	• Fibrates • Statins • Bile acid sequestrants • Nicotinic acid • Omega-3 fatty acids

apheresis is an invasive procedure, requires concomitant anticoagulation and may be available only in tertiary healthcare facilities. Table 2 describes the management of hypertriglyceridemia-induced acute pancreatitis.

Long-term management to prevent subsequent episodes includes lifestyle modification, weight loss and limiting alcohol consumption. Secondary causes of HTG like hypothyroidism and diabetes should be treated. Most patients would additionally require long-term TG-lowering agents like fibrates, nicotinic acid and/or ω-3-fatty acids.[8]

LIPID ABNORMALITIES IN CHRONIC PANCREATITIS

Chronic pancreatitis is an irreversible progressive inflammatory disorder which is characterized by acinar loss, mononuclear cell infiltration, and fibrosis. The various etiologies include alcohol consumption, tropical pancreatitis (e.g., secondary to cassava ingestion), obstructive pancreatic diseases, hereditary causes and in patients with alpha-1 anti-trypsin deficiency. Histologically, chronic pancreatitis can be classified as chronic obstructive pancreatitis, chronic calcifying pancreatitis and chronic inflammatory pancreatitis.[10]

Chronic pancreatitis is very commonly associated with EPI which manifests itself with fat malabsorption leading commonly to symptoms of steatorrhea (greasy large volume, foul smelling stools which are difficult to flush), loss of weight, and abdominal bloating or discomfort. Patients may reduce fat intake to modify and reduce symptoms. Clinically, patients may be noted to have edema, anemia, bone pains, and proximal muscle weakness (due to vitamin D deficiency), neurological manifestation and signs of coagulopathy (due to vitamin K deficiency). Establishing the diagnosis would require quantitative fecal fat collection on a high fat (100 g/day) diet over 72 hours. However, since this is cumbersome, a simple qualitative stool fat test may be used to indicate fat malabsorption. Quantification of the fecal elastase-1 (FE-1) levels may serve as an indirect marker for exocrine pancreatic function. However, FE-1 levels can only be satisfactorily quantified in well-formed stools.[4]

Although the role of lipid derangements is well established in recurrent acute pancreatitis, its role in chronic pancreatitis remains controversial and debatable. Evidences supporting its role includes several lipoprotein abnormalities (e.g., apoprotein C-II deficiency and familial lipoprotein lipase deficiency) in extended Dutch families[11,12] with heritable chronic pancreatitis. Preexisting hyperlipidemia was also found in 5 of 62 patients who were evaluated for chronic pancreatitis by DiMagno et al.[13] Despite these evidences, several other reviews link lipid abnormalities like HTG to only acute pancreatitis.[14] This may be due to the fact that recurrent acute pancreatitis dominates a majority of the spectrum of cases with genetic lipoprotein abnormalities (with poorly controlled lipid profiles) with chronic pancreatitis developing as a rare entity in this subset of patients.

Patients with EPI are treated with pancreatic enzyme replacement therapy (PERT). In addition, the underlying disease that causes EPI should also be treated. Frequent small volume feeds are recommended, and fats are not restricted in patients on adequate PERT. Difficult to digest foods like legumes should be avoided. Oral supplements of fat soluble vitamins and ω-3 fatty acids may be required.[4] Chronic pancreatitis may be associated with secondary diabetes, and many patients require insulin injectable treatment.

CHAPTER 5: Lipo-health and the Endocrine System: Pancreas

LIPOCRINOLOGY AND THE ENDOCRINE PANCREAS

The endocrine system closely interacts with adipose tissue and liver to regulate lipid and lipoprotein metabolism and the endocrine pancreatic hormones are key players in the synchronized control of intermediary metabolism. The effects of insulin and glucagon on lipid metabolism are depicted in figure 1 and summarized in table 3 and are further discussed below.

Effect of Insulin on Lipid Metabolism

Insulin regulates key enzymes involved in lipid and lipoprotein metabolism to inhibit lipolysis and increase lipogenesis. The effects of insulin on lipid metabolism are mediated by an increase in glucose uptake by adipocytes due to recruitment of glucose transporter-4 (GLUT-4) on the adipocyte cell surface. Glycolysis is also increased, and this leads to glucose being used as a primary fuel source, thereby, sparing lipids.[15] Intracellular glucose can be converted to alpha-glycerol, the active form of glycerol, via glycerol-3-phosphate in the glycolytic pathway and this effect is regulated by insulin. Glycerol combines with FFAs to form TGs with resultant increase in lipogenesis.

In addition, insulin directly regulates the activity of various lipases including lipoprotein lipase and hormone-sensitive lipase. The activity of lipoprotein lipase enzyme, that is present in the endothelium, is increased by insulin. Lipoprotein lipase causes hydrolysis of TGs within VLDL and chylomicrons to release fatty acids and glycerol. These are then taken up by adipocytes and converted back to TGs and stored in adipose tissue. At the same time, insulin inhibits the activity of hormone-sensitive lipase which controls the breakdown of intra-adipocyte TGs, and therefore, decreases

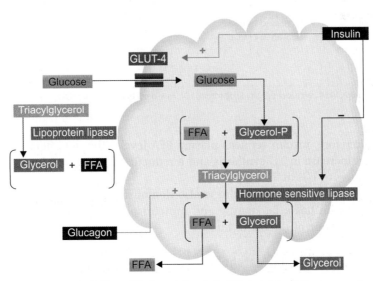

GLUT-4, glucose transporter-4; Glycerol-P, glycerol phosphate; FFA, free fatty acids.

FIG. 1: Effect of insulin and glucagon on adipocytes and lipid metabolism. The figure summarizes the effect of pancreatic hormones, insulin and glucagon at the level of the adipocytes.

SECTION 1: Lipids in Endocrinology

TABLE 3 Role of insulin and glucagon in lipid metabolism

	Function	Effect of insulin	Effect of glucagon
Hormone-sensitive lipase	• Present within adipocytes • Causes hydrolysis of triglycerides into free fatty acids and glycerol • Involved in mobilization of stored fats for energy requirements	• Decreased activity, with reduced lipolysis and reduced concentration of FFAs • Reduced fatty acid oxidation and ketone body production	• Increased activity • Increased secretion of FFAs from adipocytes into circulation • Increased fatty acid oxidation and ketone body production
Lipoprotein lipase	• Present in endothelium in adipose tissue, skeletal muscle and heart • Hydrolysis of triglycerides in VLDL and chylomicrons to release fatty acids and glycerol, for uptake into cells. Converts VLDL to IDL and then LDL	• Increased activity in adipocytes with increased uptake of FFA and glycerol into adipocytes for conversion to and storage as triglycerides. Decreased activity in the muscle	• Decreased activity in adipose tissue, increased activity in muscle and myocardium • Decreased lipogenesis
Acetyl-CoA carboxylase and fatty acid synthase	• Increased synthesis of fatty acids in adipocyte with increased lipogenesis	• Stimulated—increased lipogenesis	• Suppressed
B-oxidation/fatty acid oxidation	• Lipogenesis and fat storage	• Suppressed, reduced ketogenesis	• Increased, increase in ketone body production
LDL receptor	• Increased hepatic clearance of LDL	• Increased expression, increased LDL clearance	• Increased binding of LDL to LDLR but does not increase expression

FFAs, free fatty acids; VLDL, very low-density lipoprotein; LDL, low-density lipoprotein; LDLR, low-density lipoprotein receptor.

lipolysis. Therefore, insulin reduces plasma FFA levels. The net effect of insulin is therefore an increase in TG synthesis and a reduction in TG breakdown leading to increased stores of TGs in the adipocyte.

Similar anabolic effect of insulin is also demonstrated on protein metabolism. In general, insulin has a fat-sparing and protein-sparing effect, and increases the peripheral utilization of glucose as fuel.[15]

Effect of Glucagon on Lipid Metabolism

Glucagon has effects opposite to those of insulin on intermediary metabolism. Glucagon inhibits lipoprotein lipase and, therefore, reduces the uptake of fatty acids and glycerol by adipose tissue. It increases lipolysis in white adipose tissue by increasing the activity of hormone-sensitive lipase with resultant increase in FFA secretion from adipocytes into circulation. The FFAs are carried to skeletal and cardiac myocytes, liver, and kidney for utilization as source of energy or conversion to ketone bodies. Glucagon stimulates fatty acid oxidation and controls the production of ketone bodies that serve as an important fuel during periods of relative glucose deficiency. In addition, another important effect of glucagon is to inhibit fatty acid esterification and lipogenesis.[15]

Intravenous glucagon has been shown to reduce total lipid levels and plasma cholesterol within 30 minutes. Glucagon was also demonstrated to reduce TGs and VLDL cholesterol. Glucagon increases the binding of LDL to LDL receptor (LDLR) but does not increase the expression of LDLR.

The net effect of glucagon on lipid metabolism can be described as that of increased lipid mobilization. These effects seem to be independent of glucagon's effect on glucose homeostasis.

LIPIDS AND THE β-CELLS IN THE PANCREAS

A healthy pancreatic β-cell, in response to a rise in blood glucose secretes insulin, leading to either utilization of glucose by the peripheral tissues or storage as glycogen. The net result is a euglycemic state. In individuals with insulin resistance, the decrease in insulin sensitivity leads to abnormally larger amounts of insulin, leading to a decline in β-cell mass and β-cell adaptability.[16] This results in a gradual progressive decline in the β-cell function and ultimately manifests as T2DM.[17]

The effect of FFAs on the pancreatic β-cell and its role in insulin resistance has been extensively reported. In a state of acute FFA deprivation, there is a loss of glucose stimulated insulin secretion (GSIS), which in turn downregulates the β-cell. This process, however, is reversible. Acute exposure to high levels of FFAs, on the contrary, augments GSIS leading to a heightened secretion of insulin.[18]

In chronic exposure, there are several detrimental changes in the pancreatic β-cell. Initially there is an increase in β-cell mass, which suggests the β-cell to be in a state of neogenesis.[19] These changes were seen in Zucker nondiabetic obese rats. This compensatory hypertrophy in the β-cell explains the initial plasticity of the β-cell to adequately respond in early stages of insulin resistance. Eventually, however, this compensatory response fails to keep pace with the growing insulin resistance and culminates in frank diabetes.[20]

Insulin Resistance and the Pancreatic β-cell

Insulin resistance is the hallmark feature of T2DM and is frequently observed in obesity. In cases with chronic exposure to FFAs, there exists both β-cell dysfunction as well as impaired insulin sensitivity, and ultimately cellular apoptosis resulting in overt diabetes mellitus.[21]

Recent models have also proposed a role for genetic susceptibility in the pathophysiology of insulin resistance. It is the binding of insulin to its tyrosine kinase-based receptors that results in the phosphorylation of its various substrates. Mutations in the insulin receptor substrate (*IRS*) genes—i.e., *IRS-1* and *IRS-2*, have been implicated in the development of insulin resistance.[22]

Another key player in the development of insulin resistance is the adipose tissue. Insulin restricts lipolysis in the adipocyte normalizing the amounts of circulating FFAs.[23] This, therefore, implies that the increased amount of circulatory FFAs in individuals with insulin resistance implicates a dysregulated form of lipolysis in the adipocyte.

The various proposed mechanisms for FFA signaling of the pancreatic β-cell include the 5' adenosine monophosphate-activated protein kinase/malonyl-CoA/long-chain acyl-CoA (LC-CoA) signaling network, the glucose-responsive TG/free fatty acid (FFA) cycling and FFA stimulation of the G protein-coupled receptor GPR40/FFAR1.[20]

Lipotoxicity and the Pancreatic β-cell

Lipotoxicity, a term coined by Unger, refers to a condition where there is an abnormal spillover of lipids into tissues apart from the adipose tissue (e.g., muscle, liver, pancreas etc.), resulting in a toxic environment for these tissues.[24] Chronic exposure to elevated levels of FFAs result in both the inhibition of insulin secretion as well as the blunting of the insulin response, culminating in the inability of the adipose tissue to effectively store TGs.[25] Elevated FFAs also impair glycogen synthesis, and downregulate GLUT-4 receptors resulting in decreased glucose transport and impaired insulin sensitivity.[26]

Lipotoxicity is also associated with organ specific insulin resistance. Several magnetic resonance studies in patients with T2DM with insulin resistance, found altered visceral fat topology and fat accumulation in various tissues, which when treated with thiazolidinediones showed improvement in insulin sensitivity.[27] Lipotoxicity, thus, seems to be an advanced state of insulin resistance. Hence, interventions targeting reduction of lipotoxicity (i.e., calorie restriction, thiazolidine-diones, glucagon-like peptide 1 analogs etc.) decrease insulin resistance, whereby potentially enhancing the life of the pancreatic β-cell.[28] In addition, lipotoxicity also acts directly to impair insulin secretion and increase β-cell apoptosis due to increased exposure of pancreatic β-cell to intracellular toxic lipid metabolites. The effects of lipotoxicity in diabetes are further discussed in the chapter on "Lipotoxicity in Diabetes."

LIPIDS AND THE ALPHA CELL IN THE PANCREAS

Alpha-cells predominantly secrete the hormone glucagon that was traditionally considered as a glucogenic hormone. Recent evidences, however, suggest its added role in lipid metabolism.[29] Glucagon influences three main members in the lipid family, i.e., nonesterified fatty acids also known as FFA, ketone bodies, and TGs. It upregulates both lipolysis and ketogenesis—increasing FFAs and ketone body formation, while downregulating the TG formation. Among these, the FFAs act as a major source of energy to muscles especially in states of stress giving glucagon a novel role of a stress hormone.[30]

In contrast to the β-cells of the pancreas, information about the effects of hyperlipidemic states on the α-cells is limited. Most research is restricted to short-term effects following exposure to palmitic acid, which results in α-cell hypersecretion.[31] This, however, is far from ideal because in physiological conditions, the α-cells are constantly exposed to various saturated and unsaturated fatty acids.

THERAPEUTIC IMPLICATIONS

Diabetes is characterized by atherogenic dyslipidemia with elevated TGs and reduced high-density lipoprotein cholesterol (HDL-C), and increased total and LDL cholesterol and is associated with high cardiovascular risk. Poorly controlled diabetes can be associated with hypertriglyceridemia, which is amenable to correction with improved glycemic control. In states of severe hypertriglyceridemia as seen in acute pancreatitis, insulin can rapidly reduce serum TGs by increasing lipoprotein lipase activity and uptake into adipocytes.

Early and intensive glycemic control and lipid management also has the potential to ameliorate glucotoxicity and lipotoxicity, and thereby to retard the progression of β-cell failure as well as improve insulin sensitivity. Several antidiabetic agents have variable effects on lipid homeostasis. The thiazolidinedione, pioglitazone, causes a redistribution of fat from visceral to subcutaneous compartment, leads to reduction in TGs and increase in HDL-C. While there is a small increase in LDL-C, the LDL particle's size is increased, making it less atherogenic. By amelioration of lipotoxicity, it has shown the potential to retard the progression of β-cell failure and has demonstrated significant glycemic durability. Glucagon-like peptide 1 agonists also reduce TGs, LDL-C and total cholesterol. However, most diabetic individuals will require lipid-lowering agents for cardiovascular risk reduction. These agents themselves may have variable effects on insulin secretion and insulin sensitivity and this is further elaborated in the chapter "Endocrine Effects of Lipid Lowering Drugs."

Glucagon as a hypolipidemic hormone has been implicated in several clinical studies among patients with hyperlipidemia. Both Amatudio et al. and Aubry et al. found that glucagon therapy resulted in lower TG levels in patients with hyperlipidemia.[32,33] Moreover, hepatic catheterization studies in patients with glucagon secreting tumors have also found decreased levels of hepatic TG production.[34] The various proposed mechanisms for lowering TG levels include oxidation of fatty acids to ketones, depressing de novo synthesis of fatty acids from acetyl coenzyme A and inhibiting synthesis/secretion of lipoproteins.[35] With TGs being implicated in the pathogenesis of several metabolic conditions including insulin resistance, the evidence for glucagon as a hypolipidemic hormone is promising.[36] Further research is still required to understand its role with various other stress hormones.

CONCLUSION

The pancreas with its exocrine and endocrine components is deeply intertwined in various lipid related issues. Clinical entities (e.g., T1DM and T2DM, lipoprotein abnormalities, alcoholism, etc.) associated with hyperlipidemic states have clear implications in various diseases of the exocrine and endocrine pancreas. Hyperlipidemic states also have definitive associations in the structure and functioning of the endocrine pancreas. The understanding of β-cell physiology in relation to elevated FFAs is pivotal in insulin resistance and lipotoxicity. The clinical implications of glucagon as a hypolipidemic hormone requires further research.

REFERENCES

1. Extenman C, Chaikoff IL, Montgomery ML. The role of the external secretion of the pancreas in lipid metabolism. The influence of daily ingestion of pancreatic juice upon the level of blood lipids in completely depancreatized and duct-ligated dogs maintained with insulin. J Biol Chem. 1941;137:699-706.
2. Hegyi P, Petersen OH. The exocrine pancreas: The acinar-ductal tango in physiology and pathophysiology. In: Reviews of physiology, biochemistry and pharmacology, Vol 165. Springer; 2013. p. 1-30.
3. Pallagi P, Hegyi P, Rakonczay Jr Z. The physiology and pathophysiology of pancreatic ductal secretion: The background for clinicians. Pancreas. 2015;44(8):1211-33.
4. Alkaade S, Vareedayah AA. A primer on exocrine pancreatic insufficiency, fat malabsorption, and fatty acid abnormalities. Am J Manag Care. 2017;23(12 Suppl):S203-9.
5. Pejic RN, Lee DT. Hypertriglyceridemia. J Am Board Fam Med. 2006;19(3):310-6.
6. Yuan G, Al-Shali KZ, Hegele RA. Hypertriglyceridemia: Its etiology, effects and treatment. Can Med Assoc J. 2007;176(8):1113-20.
7. Cameron JL, Capuzzi DM, Zuidema GD, et al. Acute pancreatitis with hyperlipemia: The incidence of lipid abnormalities in acute pancreatitis. Ann Surg. 1973;177(4):483.
8. Scherer J, Singh VP, Pitchumoni CS, et al. Issues in hypertriglyceridemic pancreatitis: An update. J Clin Gastroenterol. 2014;48(3):195-203.
9. Fortson MR, Freedman SN, Webster III PD. Clinical assessment of hyperlipidemic pancreatitis. Am J Gastroenterol. 1995;90(12):2134-9.
10. Mergener K, Baillie J. Chronic pancreatitis. Lancet. 1997;350(9088):1379-85.
11. Wilson DE, Hata A, Kwong LK, et al. Mutations in exon 3 of the lipoprotein lipase gene segregating in a family with hypertriglyceridemia, pancreatitis, and non-insulin-dependent diabetes. J Clin Invest. 1993;92(1):203-11.
12. Fojo SS, Brewer HB. Hypertriglyceridaemia due to genetic defects in lipoprotein lipase and apolipoprotein C-II. J Intern Med. 1992;231(6):669-77.
13. DiMagno EP, Holtmann G. Chronic pancreatitis. Curr Opin Gastroenterol. 1991;7(5):720-5.
14. Toskes PP. Hyperlipidemic pancreatitis. Gastroenterol Clin North Am. 1990;19(4):783-91.
15. Duncan RE, Ahmadian M, Jaworski K, et al. Regulation of lipolysis in adipocytes. Annu Rev Nutr. 2007;27:79-101.
16. Pick A, Clark J, Kubstrup C, et al. Role of apoptosis in failure of beta-cell mass compensation for insulin resistance and beta-cell defects in the male Zucker diabetic fatty rat. Diabetes. 1998;47(3):358-64.
17. Stumvoll M, Tataranni PA, Stefan N, et al. Glucose allostasis. Diabetes. 2003;52(4):903-9.
18. Stein DT, Esser V, Stevenson BE, et al. Essentiality of circulating fatty acids for glucose-stimulated insulin secretion in the fasted rat. J Clin Invest. 1996;97(12):2728-35.
19. Bonner-Weir S. Islet growth and development in the adult. J Mol Endocrinol. 2000;24(3):297-302.
20. Lingohr MK, Buettner R, Rhodes CJ. Pancreatic β-cell growth and survival-a role in obesity-linked type 2 diabetes? Trends Mol Med. 2002;8(8):375-84.
21. Boden G, Chen X, Ruiz J, et al. Mechanisms of fatty acid-induced inhibition of glucose uptake. J Clin Invest. 1994;93(6):2438-46.
22. Previs SF, Withers DJ, Ren JM, et al. Contrasting effects of IRS-1 versus IRS-2 gene disruption on carbohydrate and lipid metabolism in vivo. J Biol Chem. 2000;275(50):38990-4.
23. Manganiello VC, Smith CJ, Degerman E, et al. Molecular mechanisms involved in the antilipolytic action of insulin: Phosphorylation and activation of a particulate adipocyte cAMP phosphodiesterase. In: Molecular Biology and Physiology of Insulin and Insulin-Like Growth Factors. Springer; 1991. p. 239-48.

24. Schaffer JE. Lipotoxicity: When tissues overeat. Curr Opin Lipidol. 2003;14(3):281-7.
25. Kashyap S, Belfort R, Gastaldelli A, et al. A sustained increase in plasma free fatty acids impairs insulin secretion in nondiabetic subjects genetically predisposed to develop type 2 diabetes. Diabetes. 2003;52(10):2461-74.
26. Dresner A, Laurent D, Marcucci M, et al. Effects of free fatty acids on glucose transport and IRS-1–associated phosphatidylinositol 3-kinase activity. J Clin Invest. 1999;103(2):253-9.
27. Miyazaki Y, Mahankali A, Matsuda M, et al. Effect of pioglitazone on abdominal fat distribution and insulin sensitivity in type 2 diabetic patients. J Clin Endocrinol Metab. 2002;87(6):2784-91.
28. DeFronzo RA. Insulin resistance, lipotoxicity, type 2 diabetes and atherosclerosis: The missing links. The Claude Bernard Lecture 2009. Diabetologia. 2010;53(7):1270-87.
29. Sherwin RS, Fisher M, Hendler R, et al. Hyperglucagonemia and blood glucose regulation in normal, obese and diabetic subjects. N Engl J Med. 1976;294(9):455-61.
30. Schade DS, Woodside W, Eaton RP. The role of glucagon in the regulation of plasma lipids. Metabolism. 1979;28(8):874-86.
31. Gremlich S, Bonny C, Waeber G, et al. Fatty acids decrease IDX-1 expression in rat pancreatic islets and reduce GLUT2, glucokinase, insulin, and somatostatin levels. J Biol Chem. 1997;272(48):30261-9.
32. Aubry F, Marcel YL, Davignon J. Effects of glucagon on plasma lipids in different types of primary hyperlipoproteinemia. Metab Clin Exp. 1974;23(3):225-38.
33. Amatuzio DS, Grande F, Wada S. Effect of glucagon on the serum lipids in essential hyperlipemia and in hypercholesterolemia. Metabolism. 1962;11:1240-9.
34. Boden G, Wilson RM, Owen OE. Effects of chronic glucagon excess on hepatic metabolism. Diabetes. 1978;27(6):643-8.
35. Eaton RP. Hypolipemic action of glucagon in experimental endogenous lipemia in the rat. J Lipid Res. 1973;14(3):312-8.
36. Grundy SM. Hypertriglyceridemia, insulin resistance, and the metabolic syndrome. Am J Cardiol. 1999;83(9):25-9.

CHAPTER 6

Lipid-health as an Aid to Clinical Decision-making in Endocrinology

Sanjay Kalra, Gagan Priya

> **ABSTRACT**
>
> Lipid and anthropometric abnormalities are a common occurrence in various endocrine and metabolic diseases. An understanding of these lipid alterations in endocrinopathies can be used to help screen, diagnose, differentiate, monitor, prognosticate, and plan treatment for endocrine disease. This chapter describes the multiple ways in which estimation of lipid levels and anthropometric parameters can be used to assist clinical decision-making in endocrinology. Knowledge of the multifaceted practical utility of these investigations will help understand the concept of lipocrinology.

INTRODUCTION

The field of endocrinology and metabolism is one of the most rapidly expanding of all medical sciences with new knowledge being accumulated with each passing year. New insight is being gained into normal physiology of metabolic health, complex interplay between various physiological systems, pathophysiological mechanisms of chronic metabolic disease and their inter-relationship with each other. Thus, it has opened a myriad of possible therapeutic approaches in endocrine and metabolic diseases. Each year, we witness the entry of newer molecules for the management of endo-metabolic disorders, with guidelines being updated to keep pace with research.

While new vistas are constantly being explored, this brings with it several challenges. One of the most important of these is to put research into appropriate clinical context and practice. The vital question is how to translate all this knowledge into good clinical sense. What does this information mean for the healthcare provider? It is one thing to understand that diabetes, hypothyroidism, Cushing's syndrome or polycystic ovary syndrome are associated with dyslipidemia and the mechanisms for the same. More importantly, how do we inculcate this information to improve routine patient care? In this chapter, we discuss how adipose tissue and lipid health indicators can assist in clinical decision-making in endocrine practice.

WHY IS LIPID HEALTH SO IMPORTANT IN ENDOCRINOLOGY?

It is being increasingly understood that metabolic health is closely inter-linked with endocrine health, as discussed in previous sections of this book. Several hormones intricately regulate adipose tissue differentiation, distribution, and function and modulate lipid and lipoprotein metabolism. Similarly, many drugs used in endocrinology have a significant impact on lipid health. Consequently, many endocrinopathies are associated with changes in body weight and fat distribution and measurable alterations in serum lipid fractions. At the same time, abnormalities in lipid metabolism can contribute to progression of endocrine disease, e.g. lipotoxicity impairs β-cell function in diabetes. Dyslipidemia also contributes to the increased risk of atherosclerotic cardiovascular disease (ASCVD) and is an important driver of morbidity and mortality in endocrine diseases.[1]

Hence, anthropometric assessment of weight, body mass index (BMI), waist circumference (WC), and fat distribution as well as laboratory evaluation of lipid fractions form an integral part of the endocrine clinic. Lipid estimation is, in fact done in most routine biochemistries in general clinical practice, to screen for dyslipidemia as a marker of ASCVD risk. An abnormal lipidogram can be an important clue to the presence of underlying endocrine disorders.

CLINICAL DIAGNOSIS

Adipose Tissue Distribution as a Clue to Diagnosis of Endocrine Disease

Overweight and obesity are rapidly increasing in modern times and are associated with significant comorbidities. The list of these comorbid conditions that are adding to the global disease burden includes diabetes, hypertension, cardiovascular disease, non-alcoholic fatty liver disease (NAFLD), polycystic ovary syndrome (PCOS), thyroid dysfunction, osteoarthritis, gout, gallstone disease, obstructive sleep apnea, and malignancies.[2] Anthropometry is one of the most important of clinical assessments and can be an important indicator of underlying endo-metabolic disease. As adipose tissue is considered as an endocrine organ, abnormal fat content and distribution should be considered an endocrine disorder with multisystemic implications. Several endocrine disorders such as diabetes, hypothyroidism, PCOS, growth hormone deficiency (GHD), hypogonadism, insulinomas, hypothalamic and pituitary diseases and genetic syndromes are also associated with weight gain. Weight gain with poor height gain, in fact, can be an important indicator of endocrine disease in the pediatric population.

Body fat distribution is an important factor to consider. Increased visceral and upper body fat is strongly associated with metabolic disorders. On the other hand, peripheral subcutaneous fat may not contribute to metabolic risk as strongly and may even be protective. Therefore, measures of central adiposity such as WC and waist hip ratio are considered more important than body weight or BMI. In addition, Asian Indians have greater insulin resistance and metabolic abnormalities at relatively lower BMI and WC as compared to Caucasians. So, the cut-offs for BMI and WC to define obesity are comparatively lower.[3] Other indicators toward underlying metabolic abnormalities in obese or overweight individuals include clinical features of insulin resistance such as acanthosis nigricans or skin tags. One of the first clinical clues to differentiate type 2 diabetes from type 1 diabetes, latent auto-immune diabetes of adults (LADA), maturity-onset diabetes (MODY), or pancreatic diabetes is presence of overweight and obesity in the former. However, it cannot be taken as an absolute differentiating feature as the prevalence of obesity in type 1 diabetes is also increasing.

In addition, several endocrine diseases can have typical patterns of fat distribution. While hypothyroid individuals have generalized weight gain, chronic glucocorticoid excess or Cushing's syndrome can be suspected in individuals with central adiposity, prominent buccal, supraclavicular, and dorsocervical fat and thin extremities. Lipodystrophies are characteristically associated with loss of body fat in specific depots and can be suspected on clinical examination of the same.[4] Congenital generalized lipodystrophy is associated with an almost complete absence of body fat in all depots at a young age, muscular appearance and signs of insulin resistance. Partial lipodystrophies may present with loss of fat from face, neck, upper extremities and trunk. Human immunodeficiency virus-associated lipodystrophy may be suspected when there is marked loss of subcutaneous fat in cheeks, upper and lower limbs. There may also be increased dorsocervical and central fat. Insulin induced lipodystrophy at the site of insulin injection in persons with diabetes is important to detect as it may lead to high glycemic variability and suboptimal glycemic control.

Serum Lipid Profile as a clue to Presence of Endocrine Disease

Lipid profile is a routine biochemistry panel that estimates the concentration of various lipid fractions, such as total cholesterol (TC), low-density lipoprotein cholesterol (LDL-C), high-density lipoprotein cholesterol (HDL-C), very low-density lipoprotein cholesterol (VLDL-C) and triglycerides in the blood. In addition, several laboratories report various other parameters such as cholesterol/HDL ratio, TC/HDL ratio, LDL/HDL ratio and non-HDL cholesterol as indicators of cardiovascular risk. Other estimates of risk may include lipoprotein (a) and apolipoprotein B (apoB). Non-HDL-C has gained widespread acceptance for risk stratification in addition to LDL-C.

An abnormal lipidogram should prompt clinical recall and assessment for secondary causes, which may include endocrine disease or drugs, as detailed in the chapter "Endovigilance in Lipid Disorders". Diabetes, obesity, metabolic syndrome, PCOS, and NAFLD are associated with atherogenic dyslipidemia, with low HDL-C, hypertriglyceridemia and raised small dense LDL. Young age at detection of dyslipidemia, marked elevations in serum lipids (TC >240 mg/dL or triglycerides >500 mg/dL), premature ASCVD along with clinical features such as xanthelasmas, xanthomas, arcus cornealis, or lipemia retinalis should raise the suspicion for familial hyperlipoproteinemias. When there is sudden onset of dyslipidemia, secondary causes such as endocrine disorders or drugs should be suspected. A good clinical history and examination can guide appropriate evaluation for endocrine disease.

Hypertriglyceridemia

It can occur in familial hyperlipidemias, diabetes, metabolic syndrome, PCOS, hypothyroidism, chronic kidney disease (CKD), Cushing's syndrome, GHD, and hypogonadism. Poor glycemic control in diabetes is typically associated with hypertriglyceridemia. Several drugs used in the endocrine clinic, including glucocorticoids, rosiglitazone, oral estrogens, tamoxifen, raloxifene, thiazides, and non-selective beta-blockers, can also cause hypertriglyceridemia.

Elevated Low-density Lipoprotein Cholesterol

The LDL-C is elevated in familial hypercholesterolemia, combined dyslipidemia, diabetes, metabolic syndrome, PCOS, hypothyroidism, hyperprolactinemia, Cushing's syndrome, acromegaly, and hypogonadism. In addition, drugs such as glucocorticoids, anabolic steroids, certain progestins, danazol, and rosiglitazone can also raise LDL-C.

Reduced High-density Lipoprotein Cholesterol

Obesity, metabolic syndrome and diabetes are characterized by low HDL-C. Low HDL-C and hypertriglyceridemia, in fact, serve as the defining criteria for metabolic syndrome. Other endocrine conditions associated with low HDL-C include GHD, acromegaly, hyperprolactinemia, and hypogonadism. Drugs such as anabolic steroids, danazol and progestins may also be associated with low HDL-C.

Therefore, if the clinician encounters dyslipidemia on routine evaluation, a clinical assessment and evaluation for endocrine or other systemic causes must be considered. This would include other routine biochemistry panels such as renal and hepatic panel, glycemic profile and thyroid functions. Specific testing for endocrine disease such as Cushing's syndrome, GHD, hypogonadism, lipodystrophy, and other relevant conditions should be guided by clinical suspicion.

Lipids in Radiological Evaluation in Endocrinology

Whole body fat composition has been assessed using several radiological modalities, including dual-energy X-ray absorptiometry, computed tomography (CT) and magnetic resonance imaging (MRI). This may assist in identification of the pattern of body fat distribution and quantification of various compartments including visceral and subcutaneous fat. Though these investigations are rarely used in clinical practice, such evaluation of adipose tissue is integral to endocrine and metabolic research. These modalities help to understand the pathophysiology of disease, and the impact of drugs on adipose tissue and metabolic dysfunction.

Interestingly, the adrenal glands are rich in their lipid content, and this has been exploited by radiologists to differentiate between benign adenomas and malignant lesions. Adrenal myelolipomas have macroscopic fat and can be easily differentiated from other tumors on non-enhanced CT of the adrenals. Adrenal adenomas have significant microscopic fat and are visible as homogenous lesions of <10 HU (Hounsefield units). However, some adenomas are lipid poor and may be difficult to differentiate from pheochromocytomas or malignant lesions. Contrast enhancement may be helpful. In addition, chemical shift MRI which is based on the difference in precision frequencies of water and fat has been found to be particularly helpful.[5] Fat causes a signal drop in chemical shift MRI and can point toward adrenal adenomas.

DIFFERENTIAL DIAGNOSIS OF ENDOCRINE DISEASES

It is difficult sometimes in the endocrine clinic to discern the etiology of a disorder on clinical symptomatology, e.g., it may be difficult to determine the type of diabetes in a young adult presenting with significant hyperglycemia. In addition to other features such as family history, obesity, signs of insulin resistance, presence or absence of ketosis, etc., presence of atherogenic dyslipidemia may point toward a diagnosis of type 2 diabetes. Individuals with type 1 diabetes or LADA, MODY and pancreatic diabetes often do not demonstrate significant lipid abnormalities.[6-8] However, this cannot be considered as an absolute differentiating feature and many persons with type 1 diabetes may also develop features of insulin resistance.[6] Additionally, it must be remembered that triglycerides may be elevated in individuals with uncontrolled blood glucose. Since the risk of other autoimmune diseases is higher in type 1 diabetes, a high TC and LDL-C in type 1 diabetes should prompt suspicion and screening for hypothyroidism. While MODY is not characteristically associated with significant insulin resistance and dyslipidemia, MODY-1 due to mutations of hepatocyte nuclear factor 4A (HNF4A) may have low apolipoproteins (apoAI, apoCIII, and apoB) and this can be a diagnostic clue.[8]

Several physiological changes in metabolism occur during pregnancy to meet the increased metabolic demand. Triglyceride levels increase in the third trimester along with a slight increase in cholesterol as well. However, these changes are not reported consistently. Presence of dyslipidemia in preconception period and early in pregnancy is associated with greater insulin resistance and higher prevalence of hyperglycemia [(gestational diabetes mellitus (GDM)] in later pregnancy and should prompt greater vigilance for the same.[9,10] On the other hand, the risk of GDM seems to be lower in lean women with high HDL-C. Thus, in early pregnancy lipid levels can be a pointer toward underlying insulin resistance and risk for GDM.

Lipid changes during pregnancy may also hint toward the type of diabetes in women detected with hyperglycemia for the first time in pregnancy. Women with pre-existing diabetes and more severe forms of GDM have more marked dyslipidemia than milder forms of GDM, with elevated triglycerides, low HDL-C, and sometimes raised LDL-C.[11] Women with pre-existing type 2 diabetes are likely to have higher triglycerides and lower HDL-C even in the first trimester, as compared to nondiabetic women, but may not exhibit significant difference in first trimester LDL-C and lipoprotein (a). Lipid profile in women with pre-existing type 1 diabetes usually does not differ from that of nondiabetic women.

Both primary and secondary hypothyroidism are associated with dyslipidemia, with elevation in LDL-C, TC/HDL ratio and LDL/HDL ratio. The lipid abnormalities improve with thyroxine replacement. However, the pattern of lipid alterations has been reported to be different. Central hypothyroidism is often associated with concomitant deficiency of other pituitary hormones including gonadotropins, growth hormone (GH) and/or cortisol that may also impact lipid profile. The most common abnormality reported in primary hypothyroidism is type IIa hyperlipidemia with elevated LDL-C, while type IIb or combined hyperlipidemia with elevation of both LDL-C and VLDL/triglycerides was more often reported in central hypothyroidism.[12] Though very little literature is available on the subject, the lipid profile may be more atherogenic in central hypothyroidism, as HDL-C is also reduced.

It may sometimes be difficult to differentiate between PCOS and premature ovarian failure (POF) in women presenting with secondary amenorrhea. The clinical indicators of insulin resistance in the former can offer a clue. Women with PCOS are more likely to have overweight/obesity, features of insulin resistance and demonstrate atherogenic dyslipidemia with raised LDL-C, raised triglycerides, raised non-HDL cholesterol and lower HDL-C.[13] Most of these changes are driven by insulin resistance and hyperandrogenism. On the other hand, women with POF are less likely to have metabolic syndrome and dyslipidemia. Over time however estrogen deprivation in untreated POF may cause increase in TC and LDL-C and increase in central obesity.[14]

Erectile dysfunction (ED) can occur due to a myriad of causes including vascular, hormonal, psychological, neurological, or drug-induced. Lipid panel estimation is mandatory in men presenting with ED. Macrovascular disease is often associated with atherogenic dyslipidemia and in such cases, ED is an important risk marker for CVD.[15] Therefore, individuals with ED and dyslipidemia should be carefully screened for ASCVD. Hypogonadism may also be associated with lipid abnormalities.

While in most cases, it is easy to diagnose primary hyperparathyroidism (HPT), it may be sometimes difficult to differentiate between primary and tertiary HPT in individuals who present with renal impairment, especially if a long-standing history of CKD is not forthcoming. Presence of lipid abnormalities associated with CKD may point towards a diagnosis of CKD-associated tertiary HPT. Chronic kidney disease is typically associated with elevated TG and low HDL-C. While LDL-C is not affected, small dense LDL increases and ApoB levels also increase.[16] The dyslipidemia worsens with decline in glomerular filtration rate. While some studies suggest that primary HPT may be associated with metabolic syndrome and mixed dyslipidemia, these changes have not been consistently reported.[17]

LIPIDS AS A PROGNOSTIC MARKER—CARDOVASCULAR RISK STRATIFICATION

Since the earliest publications of the Framingham study, it was recognized that total cholesterol is strongly associated with coronary heart disease. Hyperlipidemia is considered as one of the "traditional" risk factors for CVD which have a proven causal and not merely a statistical association with CVD. Many endocrine diseases are associated with abnormal lipid metabolism, and this is one of the major contributors to increased cardiovascular morbidity and mortality. Therefore, lipid measurement provides important information pertaining to etiopathophysiology, diagnosis, prognosis, and therapeutic choices with respect to cardiovascular risk.

Raised LDL-C has consistent association with cardiovascular risk. However, many laboratories do not measure direct LDL, but report calculated LDL-C, which may be affected by changes in triglyceride levels. Therefore, non-HDL cholesterol is now recognized as a co-primary or important secondary target in many international guidelines. At the same time, it is abundantly clear that hypertriglyceridemia and low HDL-C significantly increase the atherogenic risk. They feature as important defining criteria for metabolic syndrome. Metabolic syndrome is a constellation of pathophysiologically linked cardiometabolic risk factors including central adiposity, dyslipidemia characterized by raised triglycerides and low HDL-C, dysglycemia and hypertension.[18] Metabolic syndrome is associated with insulin resistance, adipose tissue dysfunction, chronic inflammation and endothelial dysfunction. Such individuals are at higher risk of complications including CVD, overt diabetes, CKD, NAFLD, sleep apnea, depression, osteoarthritis, and malignancies.

Therefore, dyslipidemia in endocrine disorders would be an important prognostic indicator of high cardiometabolic risk, requiring more vigilance and appropriate treatment. This is true for obesity including childhood obesity, prediabetes, diabetes, PCOS, NAFLD, hypothyroidism, Cushing's syndrome, GHD, hypogonadism, hyperaldosteronism, and other endocrine diseases.

The prevalence of dyslipidemia increases in postmenopausal women due to estrogen deficiency. There is a steady increase in total and LDL-C and lipoprotein (a). This is associated with a progressive increase in cardiovascular risk after menopause.[19] Dyslipidemia and metabolic syndrome in postmenopausal women, therefore, should be properly evaluated and adequately addressed. Late onset hypogonadism in men or "andropause" is also associated with a higher prevalence of the components of metabolic syndrome and may contribute to cardiovascular risk.[20]

DECISION-MAKING IN TREATMENT APPROACH FOR ENDOCRINE DISORDERS

Lipid profile can be an important guide to the therapeutic approach in the endocrine clinic. Lipid parameters usually improve, at least partially, with appropriate treatment of underlying endocrinopathy. Additional lipid-lowering therapy is indicated in individuals with a high cardiovascular risk.

Whether or not to Treat Mild Endocrine Dysfunction

Most endocrine diseases extend over a spectrum of mild or subclinical disease to overt full-blown endocrinopathy. Examples of this include prediabetes and overt diabetes, subclinical and overt hypothyroidism, subclinical hypercortisolism and overt Cushing's syndrome. It is often debated if the subclinical disorders should be addressed pharmacologically. The lipidogram can help guide therapy in such cases. While lifestyle modification and weight reduction are recommended in all individuals with prediabetes, those individuals who have additional cardiometabolic risk factors, including dyslipidemia should be considered for initiation of pharmacological therapy such as metformin, pioglitazone, or alpha-glucosidase inhibitors. Similarly, presence of dyslipidemia in individuals with subclinical hypothyroidism is associated with greater cardiovascular risk and these individuals may be considered for levothyroxine replacement therapy.[21]

Almost 5–20% adrenal incidentalomas may have subclinical Cushing's syndrome without the typical phenotype associated with chronic glucocorticoid excess.[22]

Presence of dyslipidemia (elevated cholesterol and triglycerides and low HDL-C) with other features of increased cardiometabolic risk may prompt surgical resection of the adenoma in addition to appropriate medical management of these risk factors.

Growth hormone deficiency in adults may be a component of combined pituitary hormone deficiency or isolated. Adult GH deficiency is associated with central adiposity, dyslipidemia, insulin resistance and increased cardiovascular risk.[23] An altered lipidogram may inform the need to treat these individuals with GH replacement therapy.

Deciding Optimal Therapeutic Choices in Endocrine Diseases

Treatment of underlying endocrine illness usually improves lipid abnormalities. However, they may not be completely ameliorated, and additional lipid-lowering drugs may be required in individuals with high cardiovascular risk. In addition, hormone-based treatments and other drugs used in endocrinology and diabetes management may themselves impact the lipid metabolism. These have been discussed in the chapter "Lipotropic Effects of Endocrine Drugs". The lipid profile should be considered when deciding appropriate pharmacotherapy.

Several antidiabetic drugs improve lipid parameters while others like rosiglitazone worsen the lipid profile. Levothyroxine replacement is associated with significant reduction in LDL-C in hypothyroid individuals, and total cholesterol was used as an indicator of adequacy of treatment long before TSH assays became standardized.

When using glucocorticoids, their impact on lipids needs to be considered. The effect of glucocorticoids on lipids depends on the dose, route of administration and underlying disease. High doses are associated with elevations in triglycerides, LDL-C and HDL-C. Therefore, low dose steroid replacement is preferable in adrenal insufficiency. Fludrocortisone has a glucocorticoid-sparing effect, and may be used if indicated.

In women, oral estradiol can cause a marked increase in triglycerides in women who already have hypertriglyceridemia, even though LDL-C and lipoprotein (a) are reduced, and should be avoided. Transdermal preparations have a less effect on lipid metabolism and are preferred. Hormone replacement therapy (HRT) in post-menopausal improves LDL-C and lipoprotein (a) levels but may worsen triglycerides, and markers of inflammation and pro-coagulation. The discontinuation of HRT results in reduced risk.[19] Lipids can therefore, be used to guide therapy in postmenopausal women. Presence of high LDL-C and metabolic syndrome increases the CHD risk with HRT. Therefore, HRT is best avoided in women with underlying dyslipidemia or metabolic syndrome.

Likewise, male hypogonadism is also associated with central obesity, insulin resistance and dyslipidemia, and testosterone replacement therapy results in metabolic improvement. However, the effect on lipids is variable. Intramuscular preparations reduce TC and LDL-C, but they also cause reduction in HDL-C. Transdermal preparations do not affect HDL-C and may be preferred in the presence of dyslipidemia.[24] In men with late onset hypogonadism (andropause), androgen replacement has not been consistently associated with improvement in lipids.[20] In fact, suprapyhsiological levels of testosterone cause an increase in LDL-C and decrease in

HDL-C. In individuals with underlying dyslipidemia, transdermal preparations may be better than oral or injectable testosterone.

Monitoring of Therapy

Changes in body weight, BMI, WC and lipid profile can be of key assistance in monitoring treatment in chronic endo-metabolic conditions, including diabetes/prediabetes, hypothyroidism, PCOS, NAFLD, Cushing's syndrome, hypogonadism, GHD, etc. Improvement in these parameters would indicate adherence to balanced medical nutrition therapy, lifestyle modification, and medications. Persistently elevated triglycerides may indicate inadequate dietary control or alcohol consumption. Hypertriglyceridemia may also be an indicator of poor glycemic control. Adequate treatment of endocrine disorders is usually associated with improvement in lipids and they can be considered as an indicator of optimization of therapy.

CONCLUSION

Lipid and lipid-related anthropometric estimations are simple, yet effective and versatile investigations. They help screen, diagnose, differentiate, monitor, prognosticate, and treat endocrine and metabolic disease. This chapter has provided an overview of the useful role of lipid assessment in endocrinology. By exploring the multifaceted links between lipid health and endocrine disease, the chapter underscores the relevance of lipocrinology in clinical practice.

REFERENCES

1. Kalra S, Priya G. Lipocrinology – the relationship between lipids and endocrine function. Drugs Context. 2018;7:212514.
2. Castro AV, Kolka CM, Kim SP, et al. Obesity, insulin resistance and comorbidities? Mechanisms of association. Arq Bras Endocrinol Metabol. 2014;58(6):600-9. Review.
3. Misra A, Shrivastava U. Obesity and dyslipidemia in South Asians. Nutrients. 2013;16;5(7):2708-33.
4. Garg A, Agarwal AK. Lipodystrophies: Disorders of adipose tissue biology. Biochim Biophys Acta. 2009;1791(6):507-13.
5. Herr K, Muglia VF, Koff WJ, et al. Imaging of the adrenal gland lesions. Radiologia Brasileira. 2014;47(4):228-39.
6. Katz M, Giani E, Laffel L. Challenges and opportunities in the management of cardiovascular risk factors in youth with type 1 diabetes: Lifestyle and beyond. Curr Diab Rep. 2015;15(12):119.
7. Ewald N, Hardt PD. Diagnosis and treatment of diabetes mellitus in chronic pancreatitis. World J Gastroenterol. 2013;19(42):7276-81.
8. Kim SH. Maturity-onset diabetes of the young: What do clinicians need to know? Diabetes Metab J. 2015;39(6):468-77.
9. Ryckman KK, Spracklen CN, Smith CJ, et al. Maternal lipid levels during pregnancy and gestational diabetes: A systematic review and meta-analysis. BJOG. 2015;122(5):643-51.
10. Li G, Kong L, Zhang L, et al. Early pregnancy maternal lipid profiles and the risk of gestational diabetes mellitus stratified for body mass index. Reprod Sci. 2015;22(6):712-7.
11. Gueuvoghlanian-Silva BY, Cordeiro FB, Lobo TF, et al. Lipid fingerprinting in mild versus severe forms of gestational diabetes mellitus. PLoS One. 2015;10(12):e0144027.
12. O'Brien T, Dinneen SF, O'Brien PC, et al. Hyperlipidemia in patients with primary and secondary hypothyroidism. Mayo Clin Proc. 1993;68(9):860-6.
13. Wild RA. Dyslipidemia in PCOS. Steroids. 2012;77(4):295-9.

14. Gulhan I, Bozkaya G, Uyar I, et al. Serum lipid levels in women with premature ovarian failure. Menopause. 2012;19(11):1231-4.
15. Rew KT, Heidelbaugh JJ. Erectile dysfunction. Am Fam Physician. 2016;94(10):820-7.
16. Tannock L. Dyslipidemia in chronic kidney disease. [Updated 2018 Jan 22]. In: De Groot LJ, Chrousos G, Dungan K, et al., editors. Endotext [Internet]. South Dartmouth (MA): MDText.com, Inc.; 2000.
17. Procopio M, Barale M, Bertaina S, et al. Cardiovascular risk and metabolic syndrome in primary hyperparathyroidism and their correlation to different clinical forms. Endocrine. 2014;47(2):581-9.
18. Mottillo S, Filion KB, Genest J, et al. The metabolic syndrome and cardiovascular risk a systematic review and meta-analysis. J Am Coll Cardiol. 2010;56(14):1113-32.
19. Howard BV, Rossouw JE. Estrogens and cardiovascular disease risk revisited: The Women's Health Initiative. Curr Opin Lipidol. 2013;24(6):493-9.
20. Schleich F, Legros JJ. Effects of androgen substitution on lipid profile in the adult and aging hypogonadal male. Eur J Endocrinol. 2004;151(4):415-24. Review.
21. Suh S, Kim DK. Subclinical hypothyroidism and cardiovascular disease. Endocrinol Metab (Seoul). 2015;30(3):246-51.
22. Zografos GN, Perysinakis I, Vassilatou E. Subclinical Cushing's syndrome: Current concepts and trends. Hormones (Athens). 2014;13(3):323-37.
23. Fukuda I, Hizuka N, Muraoka T, et al. Adult growth hormone deficiency: Current concepts. Neurol Med Chir (Tokyo). 2014;54(8):599-605.
24. Feingold K, Brinton EA, Grunfeld C. The effect of endocrine disorders on lipids and lipoproteins. In: De Groot LJ, Chrousos G, Dungan K, et al., editors. Endotext [Internet]. South Dartmouth (MA): MDText.com, Inc.; 2000-2017.

CHAPTER 7

Dyslipidemia as a Risk Factor for Atherosclerotic Cardiovascular Disease in Endocrinology

Subhodik Pramanik, Om J Lakhani

ABSTRACT

Hormones have widespread impact on lipid metabolism. Endocrinopathies such as diabetes, hypothyroidism, Cushing's syndrome, acromegaly, growth hormone deficiency, hypogonadism, hyperprolactinemia, and polycystic ovary syndrome are associated with alterations in lipid parameters. Raised total and low-density lipoprotein (LDL) cholesterol and reduced high-density lipoprotein (HDL) cholesterol are established risk factors for atherosclerotic cardiovascular disease (ASCVD). The role of elevated triglycerides in the causation of ASCVD is still unclear but growing evidence suggests that postprandial hypertriglyceridemia is associated with high cardiovascular mortality and morbidity. Dyslipidemia in endocrine disorders is often accompanied by other factors like central obesity, insulin resistance, hypertension, and hypercoagulability that significantly increase the risk of ASCVD. As expected, ASCVD is the major cause of morbidity and mortality in many endocrine disorders including diabetes, hypothyroidism, Cushing's syndrome, acromegaly and hypogonadism. Treatment of some endocrinopathies per se is associated with improvement in lipid profile and cardiovascular (CV) outcomes. Additional lipid-lowering therapy may be required to further reduce CV events; however, there is no clear guideline regarding the threshold to initiate the same in endocrinopathies apart from diabetes.

INTRODUCTION

All key hormones have varied effects on lipid and lipoprotein metabolism. Accordingly, lipid parameters are altered in states of hormone deficiency or excess. However, there is no clear correlation between level of hormone excess or deficiency and the degree of dyslipidemia. Typically, alterations in lipid parameters reported in endocrine disorders differ in published literature.[1] These differences may be due to a variety of factors such as differences in the duration and/or severity of disease, individual's genetic background, differences in environmental factors such as diet or lifestyle, the presence of confounders that can alter lipid metabolism such as

CHAPTER 7: Dyslipidemia as a Risk Factor for Atherosclerotic Cardiovascular Disease...

obesity or diabetes, and other unrecognized factors influencing the expression and manifestation of various endocrine disorders on lipid metabolism. In this chapter, the authors intend to describe the effect of different hormones on lipid metabolism and other cardiovascular risk factors, typical alteration of lipid parameters seen in various endocrine diseases and how these influence cardiovascular (CV) outcomes, especially atherosclerotic cardiovascular disease (ASCVD).

LIPID METABOLISM – ROLE IN ATHEROGENESIS

Lipids are defined as "any of a class of organic compounds that are fatty acids or their derivatives and are insoluble in water but soluble in organic solvents". Since lipids are not soluble in water, they are carried in the blood or extracellular fluid by special proteins called apoproteins. The assembled particles that contain lipids and apoproteins are called "lipoproteins". There are five major classes of lipoproteins: Low-density lipoproteins (LDL), very low-density lipoproteins (VLDL), intermediate density lipoproteins (IDL), high-density lipoproteins (HDL), and chylomicrons.

Dietary lipids are combined with chylomicrons in the intestinal mucosa and then secreted into the lymphatic system. Chylomicrons acquire apolipoprotein CII (Apo-CII) from HDL. The Apo-CII helps activate lipoprotein lipase (LPL) which breaks down triglycerides into free fatty acids (FFA) and glycerol. The FFA is taken up by the adipocytes. Once the chylomicron gives up FFA, the remnant particles are taken up by liver by endocytosis.

Endogenous lipids synthesized by the liver are secreted into circulation via VLDL. The VLDL, like its distant cousin, chylomicron, also borrows Apo-CII from HDL. The Apo-CII activates LPL and VLDL releases FFAs into adipose tissue. The remnant VLDL particle is eventually transformed to LDL which now predominantly contains cholesterol esters. Various cells of the body take up LDL via LDL-receptors. Lack of LDL receptor leads to familial hypercholesterolemia. Low density lipoprotein is oxidized and taken up by scavenger macrophages using scavenger receptor Class A, and this can lead to production of foam cells. This foam cell is deposited in the arteries producing atherosclerosis.

High-density lipoprotein is involved in reverse cholesterol transport and delivers cholesterol from foam cells in the arteries to the liver, where cholesterol is then excreted in the bile. The HDL also acts as a reservoir for various apolipoproteins like Apo-A1, ApoE, and Apo-CII.

SERUM LIPID LEVELS AS RISK FACTOR FOR ATHEROSCLEROTIC CARDIOVASCULAR DISEASE

Lipoprotein and lipid abnormalities have been recognized as a major CV risk factor. The Framingham Heart Study, the landmark study in CV risk epidemiology, identified elevated cholesterol, elevated blood pressure, and cigarette smoking as three major risk factors for coronary disease.

High Total Cholesterol as Risk Factor for Atherosclerotic Cardiovascular Disease

It is well established that total cholesterol more than or equal to 240 mg/dL is associated with two-fold increased risk of ASCVD. In a meta-analysis by Peters et al. the authors deduced that the pooled relative risk for ASCVD was 1.20 in men and 1.24 in women for every 1 mmol/L increase in total cholesterol.[2]

Elevated Low-density Lipoprotein Cholesterol as a Risk Factor for Atherosclerotic Cardiovascular Disease

Low-density lipoprotein cholesterol is an established risk factor for ASCVD. In 1987, the Helsinki heart study showed that gemfibrozil reduced the incidence of coronary artery disease (CAD) in men with dyslipidemia by reducing LDL cholesterol (LDL-C).[3] The JUPITER trial for rosuvastatin was terminated early as rosuvastatin was associated with substantial reduction in the incidence of CAD in both men and women with raised LDL-C within 2 years.[4]

Lower High-density Lipoprotein Cholesterol as a Risk Factor for Atherosclerotic Cardiovascular Disease

Despite reduction of LDL-C, some patients continue to have increased risk of CAD. This residual risk has been attributed to other factors such decreased HDL cholesterol (HDL-C) and raised triglycerides, among others. This led to the assumption that increasing the HDL-C levels would lead to reduced CV risk. In fact, the Framingham Study and other studies have established that higher HDL-C is protective.[5] Distilled data from four major clinical trials have estimated that there is a 2% reduction in CV risk for every 1 mg/dL increase in serum HDL-C. However, lipid-modifying drugs such as niacin that raise HDL-C have not demonstrated reduction in CV events or mortality. It is now understood that HDL-C consists of several sub-fractions including HDL2 and HDL3 and CV risk is related to HDL particle size and HDL function. Medications that increase HDL3 subclass in preference to HDL2 subclass may lead to more robust cardioprotective effects. However, at present there are no drugs approved for increasing the HDL levels.[5]

High Triglyceride Levels and Atherosclerotic Cardiovascular Disease Risk

The association of hypertriglyceridemia with ASCVD risk is not clearly established. Though elevated triglycerides are an important component of metabolic syndrome which in turn is an important risk factor for ASCVD, triglyceride elevation in isolation is not associated with increased risk of ASCVD. An excess of triglyceride-rich lipoproteins has been demonstrated to play a key role in the causation of atherosclerosis in metabolic syndrome and diabetes. Postprandial dysmetabolism refers to a state of increased glucose and triglyceride-containing lipoproteins in the postprandial state.[6] This postprandial hypertriglyceridemia has been associated with increased CV risk.

High Lipoprotein (a) and Atherosclerotic Cardiovascular Disease Risk

Lipoprotein (a) [Lp(a)] is an important independent risk factor for ASCVD. At present, however, there are no clinical studies which have clearly demonstrated that lowering of Lp(a) reduces the risk of ASCVD. Statins do not reduce Lp(a) levels and the only lipid-lowering agent with a clinically meaningful effect on Lp(a) includes nicotinic acid and proprotein convertase subtilisin-kexin type 9 inhibitors.

EFFECT OF HORMONES ON LIPID METABOLISM

Dyslipidemia is commonly seen in patients with various endocrine disorders.[1] In this section we explore the pathophysiological mechanisms resulting in dyslipidemia during various endocrine disorders.

Growth hormone (GH) increases lipolysis. The characteristic physiological effect of GH is a marked increase in FFA and ketone bodies in circulation after its administration. The major function of prolactin is to prepare for lactation including the ready availability of substrates such as lipids required by breast tissue for milk production.

Thyroid hormones increase the utilization of lipid substrate by mobilizing triglycerides stored in adipose tissue. They increase the expression of hepatic LDL receptors and clearance of LDL. Though, thyroid hormones per se are not found to have any lipolytic activity *in vivo*, this characteristic action of thyroid hormones might be potentially mediated by catecholamines. In contradiction to their other effects, thyroid hormones increase hepatic lipid output by enhancing the activity of the enzyme fatty acid synthase.

Glucocorticoids increase lipolysis and increase nonesterified fatty acids (NEFA) in circulation. Like thyroid hormones, glucocorticoids also enhance fatty acid synthase activity and hence increase hepatic lipid production. The actions of testosterone on lipid metabolism are somewhat opposite to the action of cortisol. Testosterone inhibits the action of LPL and reduces the uptake of triglycerides by adipocytes. However, it accentuates the action of hormone sensitive lipase and hence enhances lipolysis. Testosterone inhibits the differentiation of preadipocytes to adipocytes. Overall, testosterone reduces lipid accumulation in the adipocytes and reduces adipocyte pool.

The predominant estrogen, 17β-estradiol, is well known to have significant effect on lipid metabolism. Estradiol reduces the production of Apo B-100, while enhancing the production of Apo-AI and Apo-AII. Apolipoprotein B-100 is an important component of LDL while Apo AI and AII are components of HDL. Hence, estradiol has a favorable effect on lipid profile by enhancing HDL and reducing LDL.

DYSLIPIDEMIA IN ENDOCRINE DISEASES

Optimal levels of all these hormones are necessary to maintain lipid homeostasis. Not surprisingly, states of hormone excess as well as deficiency can cause dyslipidemia. Some of the lipid phenotypes are so characteristic that they often help in differential diagnosis of endocrinopathies. The typical alterations in lipid parameters and the underlying mechanisms are summarized in table 1. For more detailed discussion, please see chapters on "Lipo-health and the Endocrine System".

TABLE 1 Lipid alterations and the underlying mechanisms in different endocrine diseases

Endocrine diseases	Lipid parameters				Mechanism
	LDL	Triglyceride	HDL	Lp (a)	
Prolactinoma[7]	Increased	No change/increased	No change/decreased	Not known	• Direct effect of PRL • Hypoestrogenemia in females • Growth hormone deficiency due to mass effect
GH deficiency[8]	Increased	Increased	Decreased	No change	• Decrease in hepatic LDL receptor • Increase in hepatic VLDL production
Acromegaly[9]	Variable	Increased	Decreased	Increased	• Increased TG production from liver • Reduced LPL activity • Reduced reverse cholesterol transport due to decrease activity of LCAT and CETP
Overt hypothyroidism[10]	Increased	Normal to increased	Normal to increased	Increased	• Decrease in LDL receptor in liver • PCSK9 levels are increased
Subclinical hypothyroidism[10]	Normal to increased	Normal to increased	No change	Increased	• Decrease in bile acid synthesis • Increase in intestinal cholesterol absorption
Hyperthyroidism[10]	Decreased	Variable	Decreased	Decreased	• Increase in LDL receptor in liver • Decrease in PCSK9 • Increased conversion of cholesterol to bile acid • Decreased intestinal absorption of dietary cholesterol
Cushing's syndrome[11]	Increased	Increased	Variable	Increased	• Decrease hepatic LDL receptor expression • Stimulate TG and VLDL production • Increased adipose tissue lipolysis • Increased synthesis and secretion of ApoA1 (increase HDL)
Male hypogonadism[12]	Increased	Increased	Decreased	Increased	• Loss of antagonising effect of estrogen on LDL production • Decrease in hepatic lipase activity
Premature ovarian insufficiency[13]	Variable	Increased	Decreased	No change or increased	• Decrease ApoA1 • Decrease LDL clearance
Polycystic ovary syndrome[14]	Increased	Increased	Decreased	Increased	• Multifactorial hyperandrogenism, central obesity, insulin resistance, genetic factors

LDL, low-density lipoprotein; HDL, high-density lipoprotein; Lp(a), lipoprotein a; GH, growth hormone; LCAT, lecithin cholesterol acyltransferase, PCSK9, proprotein convertase subtilisin/kexin type 9; PRL, prolactin; VLDL, very low-density lipoprotein; TG, triglycerides; LPL, lipoprotein lipase; CETP, Cholesteryl ester transfer protein; ApoA1, apolipoprotein A1.

CARDIOVASCULAR DISEASES IN ENDOCRINE DISORDERS

Cardiovascular events are a leading cause of morbidity and mortality in endocrine diseases. Multiple observational studies have shown increased CV events in endocrinopathies but randomized controlled trials demonstrating an impact of therapy on CV risk are limited. Further, presence of confounders such as obesity, insulin resistance or hypertension in endocrine diseases may impact CV risk. Table 2 summarizes the evidence and possible confounders (factors other than dyslipidemia) for CV events in different endocrine diseases.

Atherosclerotic Cardiovascular Disease Risk in Diabetes

Atherosclerotic cardiovascular disease risk is the leading cause of morbidity and mortality for individuals with diabetes. Patients with type 2 diabetes have an increased prevalence of lipid abnormalities, contributing to high-risk of ASCVD. Multiple clinical trials have demonstrated the beneficial effects of pharmacologic (statin) therapy on ASCVD outcomes in subjects with and without CAD. American Diabetes Association has given clear guidelines for statin therapy for people living with diabetes.

Atherosclerotic Cardiovascular Disease Risk in Thyroid Disorders

Overt hypothyroidism has been shown to be a risk factor for atherosclerosis and CV disease. However, the effect of subclinical hypothyroidism (SCH) on CV mortality and morbidity has been inconsistent. The CV outcome studies suggest that levothyroxine treatment for SCH improves CV outcome in younger and middle age individuals and benefits have not been demonstrated in elderly (>65 years). Levothyroxine therapy effectively reduces LDL cholesterol and the magnitude of reduction is more for those with higher baseline LDL.[23] However, if lipid targets are not attained with levothyroxine alone, additional lipid-lowering therapy may be required as clinically indicated.

Atherosclerotic Cardiovascular Disease Risk in Acromegaly

The prevalence of hypertension, insulin resistance, dyslipidemia, hypertrophic cardiomyopathy, and endothelial dysfunction is increased in individuals with GH excess; however, the prevalence of CAD is unclear. Medical therapy in the form of lanreotide possibly decreases atherosclerotic burden as evidenced by reduction in carotid intima media thickness. As CV and cerebrovascular events are the primary cause of death in acromegaly, risk factors should be optimized by aggressive treatment of hypertension, diabetes mellitus, dyslipidemia, and by smoking cessation. However, there is no specific recommendation of the threshold for initiation of lipid-lowering therapy in acromegaly.

Atherosclerotic Cardiovascular Disease Risk in Polycystic Ovary Syndrome

Despite an increased prevalence of CV risk factors including hypertension, dyslipidemia, dysglycemia and obesity in women with polycystic ovary syndrome (PCOS), there are limited longitudinal studies, which are too small to detect differences

SECTION 1: Lipids in Endocrinology

TABLE 2 The evidence for increased cardiovascular risk in different endocrine diseases and possible confounders (factors other than dyslipidemia)

Endocrine diseases	Observational studies	Interventional studies	Confounders
Prolactinoma	• Increased cIMT[15] • Increased all cause and CV mortality[16]	Not available.	Obesity, insulin resistance
GH deficiency	• Increased coronary artery calcifications and cIMT[17] • Increased CV and cerebrovascular mortality	GH therapy may reduce CV mortality[18]	Central obesity, insulin resistance
Acromegaly	• Increase in CAC score and cIMT[19] • Increased risk of cardiomyopathy and arrhythmias • Increase in atherosclerotic heart disease uncertain[20]	Lanreotide therapy decreased cIMT[21]	Direct effect of GH and IGF-1 on heart, obesity, insulin resistance, hypertension
Hypothyroidism	• Overt hypothyroidism is associated with increased CV mortality. • SCH is associated with small increase in CV events, especially in young and those having TSH >10 mIU/L[22]	UK database suggests improvement of CV outcome in SCH for those with age 40–70 years[23]	Obesity, insulin resistance.
Hyperthyroidism	• Increased risk of total and CAD mortality and incident AF, especially with TSH ≤ 0.10 mIU/L and in elderly[24]	Not available.	Direct effect of T4 on cardiac muscle
Cushing's Syndrome	• Increased cIMT and CAC score[25,26] • Increased CV mortality[27]	With remission, increased mortality risk remains, but is reduced compared to persistent disease[27]	Central obesity, diabetes, hypertension, hypercoagulability
Male hypogonadism	• CV diseases are more common[28]	Testosterone therapy does not reduce CV outcome[28]	Obesity, metabolic syndrome, diabetes
Premature ovarian insufficiency	• Small increase in CV disease and mortality[29]	Not available	Obesity
Polycystic ovary syndrome	• Increased cIMT[30] • Significant increased risk for CV disease[31]	Not available	Central obesity, insulin resistance, hypertension, hyperandrogenemia

AF, atrial fibrillation; CAC, coronary artery calcium; cIMT, carotid intima-media thickness; CV, cardiovascular; GH, growth hormone; IGF-1, insulin-like growth factor 1; SCH, subclinical hypothyroidism; TSH, thyroid stimulating hormone; CAD, coronary artery disease.

in event rates. Nevertheless, epidemiological data point to increased CV risk in women with stigmata of PCOS. Although, statins have been shown to reduce serum testosterone level in PCOS women, clinical benefits are not very evident. Endocrine Society Guidelines suggested that until additional studies demonstrate a clear risk-benefit ratio favoring statin therapy for other aspects of PCOS, statins should only be used in women with PCOS who meet current indications for statin treatment for non-PCOS individuals.[33]

Atherosclerotic Cardiovascular Disease Risk in Cushing's Syndrome

Patients with Cushing's syndrome have a higher mortality rate than age and gender matched controls, which is mostly due to an increased risk of CV disease. Interestingly, this increased mortality risk remains even after remission of Cushing's syndrome; although, it is reduced compared to persistent disease. The ASCVD in Cushing's syndrome is multifactorial as this condition is associated with central obesity, diabetes, insulin resistance, hypercoagulability, and hypertension in addition to dyslipidemia, all of which contribute to increased risk. The indications of lipid-lowering therapy are similar to those for general population. However, atorvastatin should be used with caution in patients with Cushing's syndrome who are being treated with ketoconazole as the latter inhibits hepatic cytochrome P450 enzyme, leading to increased plasma concentration of atorvastatin and thus risk of myotoxicity.

Atherosclerotic Cardiovascular Disease Risk in Male Hypogonadism

Longitudinal studies have shown that CV disease occurs more frequently in subjects with low testosterone levels. Whether the low testosterone is causative or a biomarker of poor cardiovascular health (e.g., obesity, metabolic syndrome, diabetes) is not conclusively known. Trial of testosterone therapy in hypogonadal men has shown to be either beneficial or neutral, especially when used in patients with pre-existing CV conditions.

CONCLUSION

Alteration of lipid parameters are well documented in prolactinoma, GH deficiency, acromegaly, hypothyroidism, Cushing's syndrome, male hypogonadism and PCOS. Along with other factors like central obesity, insulin resistance, hypertension, and hypercoagulability, dyslipidemia contributes to the increased risk of ASCVD in these conditions. The ASCVD remains the leading cause of mortality and morbidity in many endocrine disorders including diabetes, Cushing's syndrome, acromegaly and hypogonadism. However, prospective studies showing impact of dyslipidemia control on CV outcome are lacking for most endocrinopathies other than diabetes. Further studies evaluating the role of lipid-lowering therapy in reducing CV burden in endocrine disorders are required. Until then, lipid-lowering therapy may be initiated based on assessment of underlying CV risk along with primary treatment of the endocrine disease state.

SECTION 1: Lipids in Endocrinology

REFERENCES

1. Feingold K, Brinton EA, Grunfeld C. The Effect of Endocrine Disorders on Lipids and Lipoproteins. 2017 Feb 24. In: De Groot LJ, Chrousos G, Dungan K, et al., editors. Endotext [Internet]. South Dartmouth (MA): MDText.com, Inc.; 2000.
2. Peters SA, Singhateh Y, Mackay D, et al. Total cholesterol as a risk factor for coronary heart disease and stroke in women compared with men: A systematic review and meta-analysis. Atherosclerosis. 2016;248:123-31.
3. Frick MH, Elo O, Haapa K, et al. Helsinki Heart Study: Primary-prevention trial with gemfibrozil in middle-aged men with dyslipidemia. Safety of treatment, changes in risk factors, and incidence of coronary heart disease. N Engl J Med. 1987;317(20):1237-45.
4. Ridker PM, Danielson E, Fonseca FA, et al, JUPITER Study Group. Rosuvastatin to prevent vascular events in men and women with elevated C-reactive protein. N Engl J Med. 2008;359(21):2195-207.
5. Woudberg NJ, Pedretti S, Lecour S, et al. Pharmacological intervention to modulate HDL: What do we target? Front Pharmacol. 2018;8:989.
6. Pappas C, Kandaraki EA, Tsirona S, et al. Postprandial dysmetabolism: Too early or too late? Hormones (Athens). 2016;15(3):321-44.
7. Ling C, Svensson L, Odén B, et al. Identification of functional prolactin (PRL) receptor gene expression: PRL inhibits lipoprotein lipase activity in human white adipose tissue. J Clin Endocrinol Metab. 2003;88(4):1804-8.
8. Cummings MH, Christ E, Umpleby AM, et al. Abnormalities of very low density lipoprotein apolipoprotein B-100 metabolism contribute to the dyslipidaemia of adult growth hormone deficiency. J Clin Endocrinol Metab. 1997;82(6):2010-3.
9. Beentjes JA, van Tol A, Sluiter WJ, et al. Low plasma lecithin: Cholesterol acyltransferase and lipid transfer protein activities in growth hormone deficient and acromegalic men: Role in altered high density lipoproteins. Atherosclerosis. 2000;153(2):491-8.
10. Duntas LH, Brenta G. The effect of thyroid disorders on lipid levels and metabolism. Med Clin North Am. 2012;96(2):269-81.
11. Taskinen MR, Nikkilä EA, Pelkonen R, et al. Plasma lipoproteins, lipolytic enzymes, and very low density lipoprotein triglyceride turnover in Cushing's syndrome. J Clin Endocrinol Metab. 1983;57(3):619-26.
12. Sorva R, Kuusi T, Taskinen MR, et al. Testosterone substitution increases the activity of lipoprotein lipase and hepatic lipase in hypogonadal males. Atherosclerosis. 1988;69(2-3):191-7.
13. Campos H, Walsh BW, Judge H, et al. Effect of estrogen on very low density lipoprotein and low density lipoprotein subclass metabolism in postmenopausal women. J Clin Endocrinol Metab. 1997;82(12):3955-63.
14. Kim JJ, Choi YM. Dyslipidemia in women with polycystic ovary syndrome. Obstet Gynecol Sci. 2013;56(3):137-42.
15. Arslan MS, Topaloglu O, Sahin M, et al. Preclinical atherosclerosis in patients with prolactinoma. Endocr Pract. 2014;20(5):447-51.
16. Haring R, Friedrich N, Völzke H, et al. Positive association of serum prolactin concentrations with all-cause and cardiovascular mortality. Eur Heart J. 2014;35(18):1215-21.
17. Murray RD, Wieringa G, Lawrance JA, et al. Partial growth hormone deficiency is associated with an adverse cardiovascular risk profile and increased carotid intima-medial thickness. Clin Endocrinol (Oxf). 2010;73(4):508-15.
18. Holmer H, Svensson J, Rylander L, et al. Nonfatal stroke, cardiac disease, and diabetes mellitus in hypopituitary patients on hormone replacement including growth hormone. J Clin Endocrinol Metab. 2007;92(9):3560-7.
19. Colao A, Spiezia S, Cerbone G, et al. Increased arterial intima-media thickness by B-M mode echodoppler ultrasonography in acromegaly. Clin Endocrinol (Oxf). 2001;54(4):515-24.
20. Mosca S, Paolillo S, Colao A, et al. Cardiovascular involvement in patients affected by acromegaly: An appraisal. Int J Cardiol. 2013;167(5):1712-8.

21. Colao A, Marzullo P, Lombardi G. Effect of a six-month treatment with lanreotide on cardiovascular risk factors and arterial intima-media thickness in patients with acromegaly. Eur J Endocrinol. 2002;146(3):303-9.
22. Ochs N, Auer R, Bauer DC, et al. Meta-analysis: Subclinical thyroid dysfunction and the risk for coronary heart disease and mortality. Ann Intern Med. 2008;148(11):832-45.
23. Razvi S, Weaver JU, Butler TJ, et al. Levothyroxine treatment of subclinical hypothyroidism, fatal and nonfatal cardiovascular events, and mortality. Arch Intern Med. 2012;172(10):811-7.
24. Collet TH, Gussekloo J, Bauer DC, et al; Thyroid Studies Collaboration. Subclinical hyperthyroidism and the risk of coronary heart disease and mortality. Arch Intern Med. 2012;172(10):799-809.
25. Faggiano A, Pivonello R, Spiezia S, et al. Cardiovascular risk factors and common carotid artery caliber and stiffness in patients with Cushing's disease during active disease and 1 year after disease remission. J Clin Endocrinol Metab. 2003;88(6):2527-33.
26. Neary NM, Booker OJ, Abel BS, et al. Hypercortisolism is associated with increased coronary arterial atherosclerosis: Analysis of noninvasive coronary angiography using multidetector computerized tomography. J Clin Endocrinol Metab. 2013;98(5):2045-52.
27. Clayton RN, Jones PW, Reulen RC, et al. Mortality in patients with Cushing's disease more than 10 years after remission: A multicentre, multinational, retrospective cohort study. Lancet Diabetes Endocrinol. 2016;4(7):569-76.
28. Dixit KCS, Wu J, Smith LB, et al. Androgens and Coronary Artery Disease. 2015 Jul 15. In: De Groot LJ, Chrousos G, Dungan K, et al., editors. Endotext [Internet]. South Dartmouth (MA): MDText. com, Inc.; 2000.
29. Atsma F, Bartelink ML, Grobbee DE, et al. Postmenopausal status and early menopause as independent risk factors for cardiovascular disease: A meta-analysis. Menopause. 2006;13(2):265-79.
30. Vural B, Caliskan E, Turkoz E, et al. Evaluation of metabolic syndrome frequency and premature carotid atherosclerosis in young women with polycystic ovary syndrome. Hum Reprod. 2005;20(9):2409-13.
31. Zhao L, Zhu Z, Lou H, et al. Polycystic ovary syndrome (PCOS) and the risk of coronary heart disease (CHD): A meta-analysis. Oncotarget. 2016;7(23):33715-21.
32. American Diabetes Association. 9. Cardiovascular Disease and Risk Management. Diabetes Care. 2017;40(Suppl 1):S75-S87.
33. Legro RS, Arslanian SA, Ehrmann DA, et al. Endocrine Society. Diagnosis and treatment of polycystic ovary syndrome: An Endocrine Society clinical practice guideline. J Clin Endocrinol Metab. 2013;98(12):4565-92.

SECTION 2

Endocrine Aspects of Lipidology

CHAPTER 8

Adipose Tissue as an Endocrine Organ

Lakshmana P Nandhini, Ankush Desai, Jayaprakash Sahoo

ABSTRACT

The adipose tissue was viewed as an inert storage tissue till a couple of decades ago. The isolation of various adipokines as well as the identification of brown adipose tissue in adults has brought a paradigm change in our understanding of adipose tissue in health and disease. The next decade will involve further basic research to complete this understanding of adipose tissue as an endocrine organ and clinical research to demonstrate therapeutic potential of some of these adipokines, directly or indirectly.

INTRODUCTION

Adipose tissue was for a long time considered as an inert storage organ of triglycerides. This idea has been revamped by the identification of unique adipose deposits in the body like brown/beige adipose tissue, the discovery of the signaling molecules secreted by adipocytes, called "adipocytokines," and the identification of several enzymes expressed in adipose tissue that have a role in hormone and metabolic pathways. The protean roles adipose tissue plays in regulating the function of other organ systems and metabolism in the body qualify it as an endocrine organ.[1] Adipose tissue dysfunction or adiposopathy is recognized as an important pathophysiological factor in the causation of obesity, metabolic syndrome, diabetes, cardiovascular disease, and nonalcoholic fatty liver disease. At the other end of the spectrum, lipodystrophies, characterized by generalized or selective loss of adipose tissue depots, are also associated with significant insulin resistance, diabetes, polycystic ovary syndrome (PCOS), nonalcoholic fatty liver disease (NAFLD) and hypogonadism. This chapter aims to delineate the different types of adipose tissue deposits in the body and their regulatory role in health and disease.

TYPES OF ADIPOSE DEPOSITS

Morphologically and functionally unique deposits of adipose tissue are known to exist.[2] These include the white adipose tissue, including subcutaneous and visceral, and brown adipose tissue (BAT), bone marrow, and perivascular adipose tissue (PVAT) depots. These are further discussed below.

White Adipose Tissue

The white adipose tissue (WAT) is the largest storage sink of triglycerides and performs distinct functions based on its location. Traditionally, the primary function of WAT was regarded as an energy store that provided a ready supply of fatty acids as a fuel in times of need. Lipid storage and mobilization from adipose tissue are intricately regulated by various hormonal and metabolic cues to match the energy supply and demand status of the body. Adipose tissue has a capacity to expand by cell hypertrophy and/or hyperplasia and increase its energy-buffering potential. However, in times of chronic overnutrition, a spillover of lipids can occur from the WAT into ectopic locations including internal organs. Since intracellular lipid metabolites can be toxic, this ectopic deposition and resultant lipotoxicity is implicated in the pathogenesis of organ dysfunction such as NAFLD and the progressive decline in β-cell function in type 2 diabetes mellitus (T2DM).[2] In addition, WAT secretes several adipocytokines and other factors that have local as well as systemic effects and plays a vital role in regulating metabolism.

White adipose tissue deposits can be broadly classified into subcutaneous and visceral adipose tissue (VAT). Subcutaneous fat depots include truncal (thoracic and abdominal subcutaneous fat) and peripheral (subcutaneous fat in upper and lower extremities including gluteofemoral region). Visceral adipose tissue is found around the internal organs and can be further differentiated into mesenteric, omental, peritoneal, and perirenal VAT.

The subcutaneous and visceral fat depots have characteristic anatomical and physiological differences, which are highlighted in table 1. Visceral adipose tissue is more cellular, has greater vascularity and is composed of smaller adipocytes, which are metabolically more active, more responsive to β3-adrenergic stimulation and less insulin responsive. Therefore, lipolytic activity of VAT is higher, leading to a greater flux of fatty acids into circulation.[3] In addition, it secretes proinflammatory adipokines. On the other hand, subcutaneous WAT has less number of adipocytes per gram of fat, is more sensitive to insulin, exhibits less lipolysis and more lipogenesis and primarily secretes anti-inflammatory adipokines. However, recent research suggests that the differences between subcutaneous and visceral fat are not as distinct as previously considered and differences exist even within subcutaneous fat depots between upper body and lower body.

Central obesity, characterized by increased VAT is associated with a high risk of developing metabolic syndrome, atherosclerosis and increased mortality. On the other hand, increased peripheral subcutaneous fat, especially in the gluteofemoral region is associated with enhanced insulin sensitivity. However, a higher amount of truncal fat along with inflammation and abnormal function of subcutaneous adipose tissue is increasingly being recognized as a contributing factor in insulin resistance and metabolic disorders.[4]

The difference in the functions of various WAT deposits are largely due to the differential secretion of adipokines, expression of metabolic signaling molecules,

CHAPTER 8: Adipose Tissue as an Endocrine Organ

TABLE 1 Salient characteristics of subcutaneous and visceral adipose tissue

	Subcutaneous adipose tissue	Visceral adipose tissue
Anatomical distribution	Abdomen, femoral, and gluteal regions, 80% of total body fat	Mesentry, omentum, 5–20% of total body fat
Cellular composition	Lesser adipocyte number, higher number of stromal cells per gram of adipose tissue	Greater number of adipocytes per gram of adipose tissue
Adipocytes	Larger adipocytes, greater differentiation of preadipocytes to adipocytes	Smaller adipocytes, metabolically more active
Vascularity	Less vascular	More vascular
Drainage	Systemic circulation	Liver via portal circulation
Innervation	More α-2 adrenergic receptors, antilipolytic	More β-adrenergic receptors, promote lipolysis
Lipolysis	Less lipolytic activity	More, generates more FFA for release into circulation, more responsive to adrenergic stimulation
FFA uptake and adipogenesis	Greater uptake of FFA for storage as triglycerides	Less uptake of FFA
Insulin sensitivity	More insulin sensitive	Less insulin sensitive
Thermogenesis	Greater number of beige adipocytes, higher thermogenesis	Less number of beige adipocytes
Secretory products	Higher expression of anti-inflammatory cytokines (leptin)	Higher expression of pro-inflammatory cytokines (IL-6, IL-8, MCP-1, PAI-1) and omentin, visfatin
Inflammatory activity	Less	Higher
Prognosis	Protective role	Associated with dysmetabolism, cardiovascular risk, and mortality

IL-6, interleukin-6; IL-8, interleukin-8; FFAs, free fatty acids; MCP-1, monocyte chemoattractant protein-1; PAI-1, plasminogen activator inhibitor-1.

and the degree of inflammation. Expression of micro-ribonucleic acids (m-RNAs) that regulate metabolic functions also varies with the different adipose deposits. Subcutaneous adipose tissue is also more responsive to insulin sensitizing agents like thiazolidinediones due to the increased expression of the nuclear receptors, peroxisome proliferator-activated receptor-γ-1 (PPARγ-1), and PPARγ-2, as compared to VAT.

Brown Adipose Tissue

Brown adipose tissue is highly vascularized and is characterized by the presence of abundant mitochondria and an increased expression of the uncoupling protein 1 (UCP-1). It has a high oxidative capacity, readily oxidizes fatty acids, and is involved in the generation of heat via UCP-1. It is localized in the supraclavicular, suprarenal, and paravertebral areas, as depicted in figure 1 and is responsible for nonshivering thermogenesis in the new born. It is now understood that BAT is present in adults as

SECTION 2: Endocrine Aspects of Lipidology

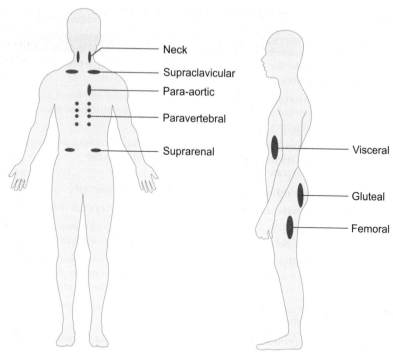

FIG. 1: Distribution of brown adipose tissue.

well. Impaired activity of the BAT has been implicated in obesity. In addition to its role in thermogenesis, BAT may have secretory functions as well. It secretes brown adipokines or batokines, including fibroblast growth factor-21 (FGF-21), interleukin-6 (IL-6), and neuregulin-4.[5] Beige or brite (brown/white) adipocytes are scattered among WAT and are morphologically similar to BAT. These cells also express UCP-1 and are thermogenic when induced by cold exposure, exercise, and β-adrenergic stimulation.

Bone Marrow Adipose Tissue

Bone marrow adipose tissue (MAT) refers to the adipocytes present within the bone marrow and acts as a secretory organ with local and systemic effects.[6] It contributes to hematopoiesis and bone remodeling and secretes adipokines like other adipose tissue deposits.[7] Marrow adipocytes influence osteoblast and osteoclast differentiation and function. Increased MAT is seen with aging and menopause and in pathological conditions like diabetes mellitus and anorexia nervosa and correlates with poor bone quantity and quality.[6] Adipokines like legumain and chemerin suppress osteoblastogenesis and subfatin impairs osteoblast differentiation and maturation.

Perivascular Adipose Tissue

Perivascular adipose tissue deposits are found around the adventitial layer of arteries and secrete several vasoactive factors, that have both endocrine and paracrine effects. The PVAT, along with the renin-angiotensin system (RAS), influences vascular functions like vascular tone, smooth muscle cell proliferation and migration, oxidative stress, and inflammatory reactions.[8] Inflammation of PVAT is associated with oxidative stress, increased macrophage infiltration, endothelial dysfunction, and activation of RAS. Chronic inflammation of the PVAT in obesity seems to independently contribute to cardiovascular dysfunction and disease.

ADIPOKINES AND KEY ENZYMES

Adipose tissue communicates with several organs and modulates their functions. This cross talk is mediated by adipokines.[9] The important WAT derived adipokines include leptin, adiponectin, resistin, retinol-binding protein 4, and visfatin. Dysfunctional adipose tissue may also secrete several proinflammatory cytokines such as tumor necrosis factor α (TNF-α), IL-6, IL-1, and IL-8.[10] "Batokines" are adipokines secreted by BAT. These include FGF-21, IL-6, and neuregulin. The functions of the adipokines are discussed in relevant sections and summarized in the tables 2 and 3 and depicted in figure 2.

TABLE 2 Adipokines and their physiological function

Adipokine	Function/significance
Adiponectin	• Promotes insulin sensitivity • Reduces hepatic glucose output • Promotes glucose uptake in peripheral tissue • Has antiatherogenic properties—inhibits adhesion of monocytes to endothelial cells and transformation of macrophages to foam cells • Improves vascular function by inducing the production of nitric oxide by endothelium • Modulates food intake and energy expenditure
Adipsin	• Promotes storage of triglycerides in adipose tissue and inhibits lipolysis
Angiotensinogen	• Precursor for Angiotensin I. Contributes to hypertension
Apelin	• Improves insulin sensitivity, fatty acid oxidation and glucose uptake in skeletal muscle
IL-6	• Decreases Insulin sensitivity • Acute phase reactant
Leptin	• Satiety signal—regulates food intake • Permissive role in signaling puberty and maintenance of reproductive function • Promotes insulin sensitivity • Promotes insulin release • Modulates T-cell function, reduced apoptosis of thymocytes
Lipocalin 2	• Acute phase reactant • Increased levels seen in obesity and associated with increased insulin resistance

Continued

Continued

Adipokine	Function/significance
Omentin	• Visceral fat deposit specific adipokine • Promotes insulin sensitivity • Suppresses TNF-α and IL-6 • Inversely related to obesity
Progranulin	• Positively associated with VAT and insulin resistance • Hyperprogranulinemia is associated with diabetic retinopathy and nephropathy • Has neuroprotective effect and its deficiency is associated with neurodegenerative disorders
Resistin	• Increases hepatic glucose production • Has proinflammatory activity • Enhances expression of VCAM-1 by endothelial cells • Elevated levels seen in obesity and T2DM
Retinol binding protein 4	• Interferes with insulin signaling in skeletal muscles • Promotes hepatic gluconeogenesis • Increases insulin resistance and occurrence of T2DM in obese individuals
TNF-α	• Contributes to insulin resistance • Mediates chronic inflammation and promotes atherosclerosis

IL-6, interleukin-6; VAT, visceral adipose; VCAM-1, vascular cell adhesion molecule-1; T2DM, type 2 diabetes mellitus; TNF-α, tumor necrosis factor-α.

TABLE 3 Batokines and their physiological function

Batokine	Function/significance
Angiopoietin-like 8	• Promotes beta cell function
FGF-21	• Induces browning of WAT • Improves beta cell function and insulin secretion
IGFBP2	• Promotes bone formation
Neuregulin	• Inhibits hepatic lipogenesis

FGF-21, fibroblast growth factor-21; IGFBP2, insulin-like growth factor-binding protein 2; WAT, white adipose tissue.

In addition, the adipose tissue also expresses key enzymes, enlisted in table 4, that are involved in energy regulation, glucose, and lipid homeostasis including hormone-sensitive lipase, lipoprotein lipase, and PPAR-γ. Several other enzymes expressed in the adipose tissue are involved in conversion, metabolism, and action of steroid hormones and include aromatase, 11β-hydroxysteroid dehydrogenases (11β-HSD) 1 and 2, 5α-reductase, and sulfatase.[11] Thus, adipose tissue acts in synchrony with other hormones in the regulation of endocrine and metabolic homeostasis.[12]

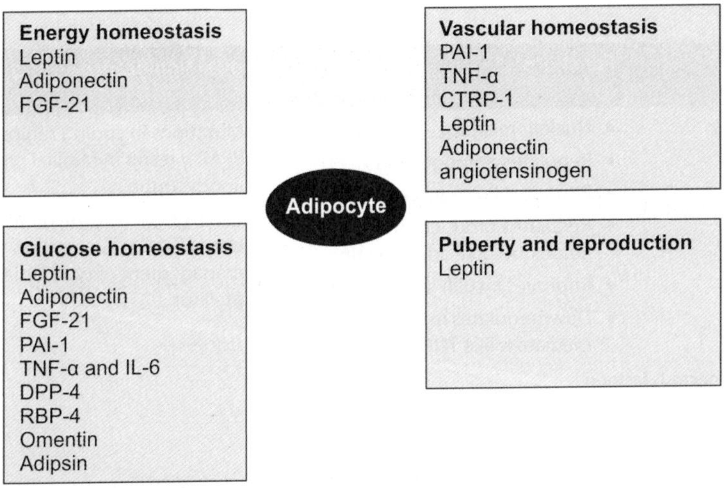

CHAPTER 8: Adipose Tissue as an Endocrine Organ

Adipocyte

Energy homeostasis
Leptin
Adiponectin
FGF-21

Vascular homeostasis
PAI-1
TNF-α
CTRP-1
Leptin
Adiponectin
angiotensinogen

Glucose homeostasis
Leptin
Adiponectin
FGF-21
PAI-1
TNF-α and IL-6
DPP-4
RBP-4
Omentin
Adipsin

Puberty and reproduction
Leptin

CTRP-1, C1q/TNF-related protein; DPP-4, dipeptidyl peptidase 4; FGF-21, fibroblast growth factor 21; PAI-1, plasminogen activator inhibitor 1; RBP-4, retinol binding protein 4; TNF-α, tumor necrosis factor-α.

FIG. 2: Adipokines secreted by adipose tissue and their physiological functions.

TABLE 4 Enzymes/receptors expressed by adipocytes

Enzymes expressed	Functions	Clinical significance
Steroid sulfatase	• Converts dehydro-epiandrosterone sulfate and dehydroepiandrosterone to estrone	• White adipose tissue (WAT) is the predominant source of estrogens in post-menopausal women
Aromatase	• Converts androstenedione to estrone and testosterone to estradiol	• Increased incidence of gynecomastia among obese men • Increased circulating and local estrogen levels contribute to development of breast cancer in obese women
11-β hydroxysteroid dehydrogenase (11-β HSD) type 1	• Converts the inactive steroid metabolite cortisone to its active form, cortisol	• Increased 11-β HSD expression in the visceral WAT contributes to increase in local levels of cortisol which mediates insulin resistance and metabolic syndrome
Lipoprotein lipase	• Hydrolyses chylomicrons and very low-density lipoprotein synthesized by liver to provide non-esterified fatty acids for storage in adipose tissue	–
Hormone sensitive lipase (HSL)	• Promotes lipolysis of triglycerides in adipose tissue • Epinephrine, norepinephrine, and glucagon promote HSL while insulin antagonizes it	–

Continued

SECTION 2: Endocrine Aspects of Lipidology

Continued

Enzymes expressed	Functions	Clinical significance
Peroxisome proliferator-activated receptor-γ (PPAR-γ)	• Nuclear receptor • Regulates adipogenesis • Promotes lipid storage • Regulates production of adipokines like adiponectin • Improves insulin sensitivity • Downregulates inflammatory mediators like TNF-α	• Mutations in coding region of PPAR-γ result in familial partial lipodystrophy • PPAR-γ agonists, the glitazone class of drugs, are used in the management of type 2 diabetes mellitus

TNF-α, tumor necrosis factor-α.

Role of Adipose Tissue in Thermogenesis

Adipose tissue plays an important role in thermoregulation. On exposure to cold, β-adrenergic receptors expressed by WAT and BAT are activated. This promotes lipolysis and flux of fatty acids from the WAT to BAT. In addition, expression of UCP-1 and mitochondrial genes in the BAT is activated. Increased expression of UCP-1 favors dissipation of energy as heat over ATP production. Thermogenically activated BAT releases large amounts of FGF-21 which acts in an autocrine manner to promote metabolism in BAT.[5] Presence of BAT in adults, in the interscapular region, has been linked with lower weight and total fat content and a decreased risk of diabetes.[13]

While WAT per se has sparse mitochondrial activity, recent research suggests that there exists plasticity among various adipose tissue deposits. The oxidative activity of WAT may be increased in response to certain physiological or pharmacological stimuli, leading to increased fatty acid oxidation, and thermogenesis. This has been referred to as "browning" of WAT. These intermediate "beige" adipocytes have been demonstrated in the subcutaneous adipose tissue deposits.[13] Peroxisome proliferator-activated receptor-γ and β3-adrenergic receptors seem to play a role in this plasticity.[2] Thyroid hormones also promote thermogenesis by activating BAT. An increased understanding of this plasticity of adipose tissue and the contributing factors may open new therapeutic avenues in the management of obesity and T2DM.[13]

ROLE OF ADIPOSE TISSUE IN FOOD INTAKE

Leptin, the most abundant adipokine secreted by the white adipose tissue, plays a crucial role in energy homeostasis along with ghrelin, that is secreted from the gastrointestinal tract. Ghrelin increases appetite, gastric acid secretion and gastrointestinal motility. Food intake results in reduced secretion of ghrelin and suppression of appetite. While this effect is immediate, the effect of leptin on satiety and energy balance seems to be more long-term.[14] Leptin receptors (LEPR) are abundantly expressed in the brain and hypothalamus, where it promotes satiety by modulating other neuropeptides and reduces food intake. At the arcuate nucleus, it stimulates the release of anorexigenic peptides, pro-opiomelanocortin (POMC) and cocaine and amphetamine-regulated transcript (CART) and inhibits synthesis of orexigenic molecules, neuropeptide Y and agouti-related peptide.[12] Leptin and LEPR deficiency is associated with marked hyperphagia and rapid weight gain in infancy, with severe obesity in childhood. Leptin deficiency can be treated with subcutaneous recombinant human leptin, metreleptin. Patients with generalized lipodystrophy also demonstrate markedly low leptin levels and are responsive to metreleptin treatment. On the other hand, obesity is characterized by hyperleptinemia due to resistance to the action of leptin.

ROLE OF ADIPOSE TISSUE IN GLUCOSE HOMEOSTASIS AND INSULIN SENSITIVITY

The adipose tissue plays a fundamental role in insulin signaling and glucose homeostasis. Different fat depots may vary in their responsivity to the antilipolytic effects of insulin, with subcutaneous fat generally regarded as more insulin responsive.

Various adipokines also regulate insulin sensitivity. Leptin has a favorable effect on insulin sensitivity. Leptin improves insulin sensitivity at the peripheral tissues and in addition, mitigates the central insulin resistance that exists at the level of hypothalamus.[12]

Adiponectin also improves insulin resistance at the liver and muscle and acts in concert with leptin. Adiponectin suppresses hepatic glucose production through adenosine monophosphate-activated protein kinase (AMPK) pathway and up-regulates the expression of insulin receptor substrate-2 (IRS-2), a vital component of insulin signaling pathway. It also promotes glucose uptake at the skeletal muscles by increasing the translocation of glucose transporter-4 (GLUT-4) protein.[15] Induction of fatty acid oxidation by adiponectin leads to reduced adipose deposits in the liver and muscle, which also enhances insulin sensitivity. Brown adipose tissue-derived FGF-21 favors glucose uptake and utilization by adipose tissue and thus improves glucose and lipid levels.[12]

The adipose tissue and pancreatic beta cells communicate with and regulate each other. Leptin inhibits the synthesis and release of insulin, while insulin promotes the release of leptin from adipocytes. Disruption of this "adipoinsular" axis due to leptin resistance at the pancreatic beta cells contributes to hyperinsulinemia.[12] Leptin also attenuates the actions of incretins on insulin secretion. Fibroblast growth factor 21 improves beta cell function and survival. It protects the β-cells from glucotoxicity and lipotoxicity and cytokine induced damage.[16] On the other hand, excess release of free fatty acids from dysfunctional adipose tissue and proinflammatory cytokines result in lipotoxicity with resultant impairment of insulin secretion from the pancreatic β-cells.

ROLE OF ADIPOSE TISSUE IN PUBERTY AND REPRODUCTION

Adipose tissue and reproductive function are intricately linked. Puberty is said to be "metabolically gated " and leptin serves as an indicator of adequate energy stores in the body that are required for the function of reproduction. From a phylogenetic viewpoint, this seems logical during times of energy deprivation. Leptin plays a permissive role in signaling the onset of puberty by directly or indirectly relaying information about the metabolic state to the kisspeptin 1 (KISS1) neurons in the arcuate nucleus, the pacemaker of pubertal development.[17] Genetic mutations in genes coding for leptin and leptin receptor have been identified in patients with obesity and hypogonadotropic hypogonadism, conforming the role of leptin in pubertal development.

Maintenance of reproductive function is also regulated by leptin. Functional hypothalamic amenorrhea resulting from severe calorie restriction due to anorexia nervosa, or stress is characterized by anovulation and hypoleptinemia. Like hypoleptinemia, hyperleptinemia has also been linked to abnormalities of the hypothalamic-pituitary-gonadal axis and reduced fertility among patients with obesity and T2DM.[17] Resistance to the actions of leptin, akin to insulin resistance, has been demonstrated in obese individuals and could together contribute to the development of PCOS.

ROLE OF ADIPOSE TISSUE IN DISEASE

Obesity, Inflammation, and Metabolic syndrome

Obesity is a proinflammatory state and is characterized by an overall shift in adipokine profile from anti-inflammatory to more proinflammatory type. Chronic inflammation is particularly seen with truncal adiposity and deposition of fat in ectopic sites such as visceral organs, while lower body subcutaneous fat seems to be protective.

Tumor Necrosis Factor Alpha and Interleukin-6

Tumor necrosis factor-α and IL-6 are cytokines that play a key role in several immunological processes and diseases. Both are secreted by the WAT and their circulative levels are proportional to the fat content and hyperinsulinemia.[12] The cytokines contribute to insulin resistance through several mechanisms; directly by antagonizing insulin signaling and indirectly by suppressing the secretion of adiponectin, increasing the circulating free fatty acid levels and downregulating PPAR. Increased levels of circulating cytokines have devastating consequences like accelerated atherosclerosis and adverse cardiac outcomes. However, this is reversible with weight loss and reduction of body fat.

Plasminogen Activator Inhibitor-1

Plasminogen activator inhibitor-1 (PAI-1) is released from visceral adipocytes and vascular endothelial cells. In addition to its contribution to insulin resistance and development of type-2 diabetes in obesity, its prothrombotic activity accelerates the vascular complications of diabetes. Plasminogen activator inhibitor-1 also suppresses PPAR-γ activity, an important regulator of adipocyte differentiation.[18] Tumor necrosis factor-α induces the expression of PAI-1 and amplifies the burden of insulin resistance.

Retinol Binding Protein-4

Retinol binding protein-4 (RBP-4) is inversely related to insulin sensitivity. High levels of RBP-4 are associated with reduced glucose uptake by peripheral tissues and increased hepatic glucose output. Some studies have shown that changes in RBP-4 levels could be one of the earliest markers that signals the onset of insulin resistance and T2DM.

Dipeptidyl Peptidase-4

Dipeptidyl peptidase-4 (DPP-4) is a transmembrane glycoprotein that inactivates a variety of substrates by cleaving the N terminal dipeptides. Glucagon-like peptide-1 and gastric inhibitory polypeptide are incretins that are degraded by DPP-4. Incretins potentiate glucose-induced insulin release and impaired incretin effect is one of the several pathogenic mechanisms that underlie T2DM. Dipeptidyl peptidase-4 is also an adipokine and its expression is promoted by proinflammatory markers like TNF-α.[12] In obese and insulin resistant individuals, DDP-4 is released predominantly from the visceral adipose tissue and correlates with adipocyte size and inflammation.

Diabetes

While adipose tissue dysfunction is clearly implicated in obesity and metabolic syndrome, the associated proinflammatory state has a key role in the pathogenesis of diabetes. Abnormal expression of adipocytokines has been associated with impaired insulin signaling, insulin resistance and dysglycemia.[1] In fact, adipose tissue insulin resistance is an important component of the ominous octet in the pathophysiology of T2DM. Diabetes is associated with both glucotoxicity and lipotoxicity, that lead to further progression of diabetes. Lipotoxicity can propagate further decline in β-cell function and increase β-cell apoptosis.[16] It is now understood that adipose tissue also secretes adipokines that improve metabolism and reduce inflammation. Modulation of the adipokine profile of adipose tissue can be a therapeutic strategy in diabetes management. Thiazolidinediones act to reduce proinflammatory adipokines, reduce lipotoxicity and have been shown to have glycemic durability. Further, transplantation of healthy white adipose tissue in rodents was found to improve glycemic control.[16]

Hypertension

Obesity and metabolic syndrome are associated with systemic hypertension. While insulin resistance itself contributes to hypertension, adipose tissue furthers the risk by modulating the adrenal and local production of aldosterone.[19] Complement-C1q TNF-related protein-1 (CTRP-1), an adipokine secreted by the stromal vasculature of adipose tissue, and leptin upregulate adrenal aldosterone synthesis. In fact, a positive correlation exists between body mass index and plasma aldosterone levels in obese individuals and aldosterone levels decrease with weight reduction. Serum levels of CTRP-1 are elevated in patients with metabolic syndrome and T2DM. Elevated adipocyte-derived aldosterone has been observed in obese animals and contributes to hypertension.

Both aldosterone and glucocorticoids can act on the mineralocorticoid receptor in adipose tissue, as this tissue expresses low levels of 11β-hydroxysteroid dehydrogenase 2 (11β-HSD2) that results in increased conversion of cortisol to inactive cortisone and higher levels of 11β-HSD 1, resulting in increased conversion of cortisone to active cortisol.[20] Mineralocorticoid receptor signaling, in turn, has been implicated in increased expression of proinflammatory cytokines, chronic inflammatory state and insulin resistance, endothelial dysfunction, vascular and cardiac remodeling, hypertension, and progression of target organ damage such as cardiovascular and chronic kidney disease.[20] Mineralocorticoid receptor antagonists are useful in the management of resistant hypertension and cardiovascular risk reduction.

THERAPEUTIC IMPLICATIONS

An increased understanding of different adipose tissue depots and their endocrine functions in health and disease provides an interesting opportunity to explore newer therapies for metabolic disorders. Identification of adipokines and an understanding of their role in regulation of insulin sensitivity has opened potential avenues for treatment of obesity, insulin resistance and diabetes mellitus. Table 5 enlists some of these therapeutic possibilities which are available or underdevelopment.

Leptin deficiency and leptin receptor mutation are rare causes of monogenic obesity. Hyperphagia and reduced energy expenditure are hallmarks of leptin and leptin receptor mutations. Recombinant leptin (metreleptin) therapy successfully reduces weight and reverses metabolic derangements and hypogonadism in patients with congenital leptin deficiency. Metreleptin has also been found to be useful in patients with generalized lipodystrophy and severe cases of partial lipodystrophy.

Rodent studies have shown that administration of adiponectin can reverse insulin resistance and has antiatherogenic effects. Recombinant adiponectin and adiponectin receptor agonists are potential agents for management of obesity. Inhibitors of TNF-α have been shown to reduce insulin resistance in animal studies.[18] Pharmacological inhibition of 11β-HSD1 enzyme could be another solution to manage obesity and metabolic syndrome.

The nuclear receptor PPAR-γ regulates adipogenesis. The PPAR-γ agonists cause preferential expansion of subcutaneous adipose deposits and cause a shift of fat from VAT to subcutaneous tissue, with resultant improvement in adipokine profile. While this is associated with significant improvement in insulin sensitivity, it also results in an improved ability of adipose tissue to act as an energy buffer. Peroxisome proliferator-activated receptor-γ agonists also promote browning of white adipocytes. The net result is reduced lipotoxicity.

TABLE 5 Therapeutic implications of the endocrine role of adipose tissue

In clinical practice	Underdevelopment
• PPAR-γ agonists (thiazolidinediones) in type 2 diabetes mellitus, PCOS, NAFLD • Recombinant human leptin (metreleptin) in leptin deficiency and lipodystrophies	• Recombinant adiponectin • Adiponectin receptor agonists • Inhibitors of TNF-α • 11β-HSD 1 inhibitors • β3-adrenergic receptor agonists (mirabegron) • FGF-21 analogs • Transplantation of brown adipose tissue

11β-HSD, 11β hydroxysteroid dehydrogenase; FGF, fibroblast growth factor; NAFLD, nonalcoholic fatty liver disease; PCOS, polycystic ovary syndrome; PPAR, peroxisome proliferator-activated receptor; TNF-α, tumor necrosis factor-α.

Modulating BAT function could serve as an antiobesity tool. Cold training recruits BAT and improves metabolic function. β3-adrenergic receptor signaling stimulates lipolysis of triglycerides to increase fatty acid mobilization and transcription of UCP-1 and PGC-1α, which results in increased fatty acid oxidation. β3-adrenergic receptor agonists have been found to induce browning of adipocytes and increase their oxidative capacity in rodent models, but human studies have been disappointing so far.[2] β3-adrenergic agonists like Mirabegron that activate BAT metabolism have a promising therapeutic potential.[21]

Transplantation of BAT has been shown to promote energy expenditure, ameliorate obesity, improve insulin sensitivity and glucose uptake in skeletal muscles, and improve glucose homeostasis in mice models of obesity and diabetes.[22] Clinical trials of FGF-21 analogs have yielded significant positive effects on bodyweight reduction and dyslipidemia.

CONCLUSION

The paradigm of adipose tissue function is changing at dramatic pace as new facts are being discovered. While adipose tissue is an important storage organ for energy, it works in close harmony with the endocrine system to regulate energy metabolism, glucose, and lipid homeostasis. It is also an important endocrine organ that secretes several adipocytokines with a broad range of metabolic effects. Brown and beige adipocytes have an additional important function of thermogenesis and have been found to be active in adults as well. This knowledge has added clarity to our understanding of conditions like obesity, insulin resistance, metabolic syndrome, diabetes, cardiovascular disease, and several malignancies. The bench to bedside translation of such knowledge has exciting therapeutic potential that can transform the management of such conditions.

REFERENCES

1. Booth A, Magnuson A, Fouts J, et al. Adipose tissue: an endocrine organ playing a role in metabolic regulation. Horm Mol Biol Clin Investig. 2016;26(1):25-42.
2. Lee YH, Mottillo EP, Granneman JG. Adipose tissue plasticity from WAT to BAT and in between. Biochim Biophys Acta. 2014;1842(3):358-69.
3. Ibrahim MM. Subcutaneous and visceral adipose tissue: structural and functional differences. Obes Rev. 2010;11(1):11-8.
4. Patel P, Abate N. Role of subcutaneous adipose tissue in the pathogenesis of insulin resistance. J Obes. 2013;2013:489187.
5. Villarroya F, Cereijo R, Villarroya J, et al. Brown adipose tissue as a secretory organ. Nat Rev Endocrinol. 2017;13(1):26-35.
6. Hawkes CP, Mostoufi-Moab S. Fat-bone interaction within the bone marrow milieu: Impact on hematopoiesis and systemic energy metabolism. Bone. 2018;pii:S8756-3282(18)30119-4.
7. Sulston RJ, Cawthorn WP. Bone marrow adipose tissue as an endocrine organ: Close to the bone? Horm Mol Biol Clin Investig. 2016;28(1):21-38.
8. Agabiti-Rosei C, Paini A, De Ciuceis C, et al. Modulation of Vascular Reactivity by Perivascular Adipose Tissue (PVAT). Curr Hypertens Rep. 2018;20(5):44.
9. Luo L, Liu M. Adipose tissue in control of metabolism. J Endocrinol. 2016;231(3):R77-99.

10. Stojsavljević S, Gomerčić Palčić M, Virović Jukić L, et al. Adipokines and proinflammatory cytokines, the key mediators in the pathogenesis of nonalcoholic fatty liver disease. World J Gastroenterol. 2014;20(48):18070-91.
11. Tchernof A, Mansour MF, Pelletier M, et al. Updated survey of the steroid-converting enzymes in human adipose tissues. J Steroid Biochem Mol Biol. 2015;147:56-69.
12. Smitka K, Marešová D. Adipose tissue as an endocrine organ: An update on proinflammatory and anti-inflammatory microenvironment. Prague Med Rep. 2015;116(2):87-111.
13. Lidell ME, Betz MJ, Enerbäck S. Brown adipose tissue and its therapeutic potential. J Intern Med. 2014;276(4):364-77.
14. Farooqi IS, O'Rahilly S. 20 years of leptin: human disorders of leptin action. J Endocrinol. 2014;223(1):T63-70.
15. Fonseca-Alaniz MH, Takada J, Alonso-Vale MI, et al. Adipose tissue as an endocrine organ: From theory to practice. J Pediatr (Rio J). 2007;83(5 Suppl):S192-203.
16. Gunawardana SC. Benefits of healthy adipose tissue in the treatment of diabetes. World J Diabetes. 2014;5(4):420-30.
17. Elias CF, Purohit D. Leptin signaling and circuits in puberty and fertility. Cell Mol Life Sci. 2013;70(5):841-62.
18. Adamczak M, Wiecek A. The adipose tissue as an endocrine organ. Semin Nephrol. 2013;33(1):2-13.
19. Dinh Cat AN, Friederich-Persson M, White A, et al. Adipocytes, aldosterone and obesity-related hypertension. J Mol Endocrinol. 2016;57(1):F7-F21.
20. Williams JS, Williams GH. 50th anniversary of aldosterone. J Clin Endocrinol Metab. 2003;88(6):2364-72.
21. Cypess AM, Weiner LS, Roberts-Toler C, et al. Activation of human brown adipose tissue by a β3-adrenergic receptor agonist. Cell Metab. 2015;21(1):33-8.
22. Tran TT, Kahn CR. Transplantation of adipose tissue and stem cells: Role in metabolism and disease. Nat Rev Endocrinol. 2010;6(4):195-213.

CHAPTER 9

Lipotoxicity and Diabetes Mellitus

Sameer Aggarwal, Jaikrit Bhutani

> **ABSTRACT**
>
> The parallel epidemic of obesity and diabetes suggests a close relationship between them. With the available evidence, adipose tissue is being considered as an endocrine organ, besides merely being a fat storage tissue. Most metabolic disorders, including obesity and diabetes are linked to dysfunctional adipocytes, leading to hypertrophy, macrophage infiltration, impaired insulin signaling and eventually insulin resistance. The underlying mechanisms include secretion of inflammatory adipokines, and free fatty acids causing ectopic fat deposition and lipotoxicity in muscle, liver, and pancreatic β-cells. This chapter briefly describes the close association of the profound effects of lipotoxicity on glucose homeostasis.

INTRODUCTION

The pathogenesis of type 2 diabetes mellitus (T2DM) revolves around defects in insulin secretion and action. Defects in insulin secretion pattern and hyperinsulinemia have been well identified in patients who develop obesity or hyperglycemia and their nondiabetic first-degree relatives. Reduced cellular (adipocyte) uptake of glucose and its abnormal metabolism in muscle and liver have been clearly identified in T2DM patients. The course from insulin resistance to symptomatic diabetes is accelerated by obesity; however, the underlying mechanisms and relevant treatment options remain less understood.

Chronic hyperglycemia has a deleterious effect on β-cell function and survival and insulin action which further contributes to hyperglycemia and leads to a relentless decline in β-cell function. This concept is referred to as glucotoxicity. However, another equally important contributor in the pathogenesis of diabetes seems to be abnormal lipid metabolism. Unger originally coined the term "lipotoxicity" to explain the deleterious effects of adipose tissue dysfunction and abnormal lipid metabolism on insulin secretion and action. The concept of lipotoxicity has since been expanded as it was demonstrated that adipose tissue dysfunction led to a state of chronic

SECTION 2: Endocrine Aspects of Lipidology

lipid overload and its accumulation in adipose as well as nonadipose tissues such as pancreas, liver, skeletal muscle, heart, and kidneys. The resultant chronic excess of free fatty acids (FFAs) disrupts key intracellular signaling pathways causing cell dysfunction and cell apoptosis. These alterations are believed to have a key role in pathophysiology of diabetes progression and development of complications.[1]

In this chapter, we emphasize on research pertaining to lipotoxicity in diabetes, and the altered adipocyte biology and its adverse effects on glucose homeostasis. The effect of increased circulating FFAs and lipotoxicity leading to pancreatic β-cell dysfunction in humans are discussed in detail. We also review suggested and future therapies for early intervention for obesity and related conditions in populations at high risk for developing T2DM.

BURDEN OF TYPE 2 DIABETES MELLITUS AND OBESITY

The global burden of diabetes is rising rapidly with marked escalation of prevalence in the South Asian countries, especially India. The recent data from International Diabetes Federation, India, reports that around 69.2 million people have T2DM and it is projected that this number will go up to 123.5 million by 2040. Also, a recent study reported a prediabetes prevalence of 6–15%, which is almost double the prevalence of diabetes in India.[2] These numbers clearly indicate that diabetes is a problem of major public health importance, which is associated with significant morbidity, healthcare costs, and mortality risk.

A major risk factor for the rising incidence of T2DM is the parallel obesity epidemic. This has been shown to be linked with higher socioeconomic status, physical inactivity, and social urbanization in India. The prevalence of generalized obesity [body mass index (BMI) ≥25 kg/m^2] in India ranges from 11.8 to 31.3% according to a recent study. It also reported that around 7.8–15.2% were overweight (BMI ≥23 kg/m^2 but <25 kg/m^2).[3] An extrapolation of these figures to entire India estimated that around 135 million people may have generalized obesity. Another burgeoning issue is the rising prevalence of childhood obesity that has an even more deleterious impact on long-term cardiometabolic health. The pooled estimated prevalence of childhood overweight and obesity in India is 19.3%.[4] In a large cohort of school going children, it was observed that each 1 unit increase in BMI increased the risk of coronary artery disease by 15%.[5] Another 24-year follow-up study of 4,857 nondiabetic American-Indian children reported that there was a 2.3 times increased risk of premature death as adults in those who had childhood obesity.[6]

LIPOPHENOTYPE IN DIABETES

The characteristic lipid abnormalities associated with diabetes have often been referred to as "atherogenic dyslipidemia". According to the Framingham Study, 9% of diabetic men, and 15% of diabetic women had elevated low density lipoprotein-cholesterol (LDL-C) levels, almost comparable to 11% and 16% of nondiabetic controls.[7] Similar findings from the United States National Health and Nutritional Examination Survey, 1999–2000 were reported, where 25.3% of diabetics and 24.3% nondiabetics had increased LDL-C.[8]

Although, the lipophenotype in terms of LDL-C of diabetic individuals is comparable to general population, the number and density of LDL particles is increased in diabetic individuals with high triglyceride levels. This excess of small dense LDL and increased particle number along with reduced high density lipoprotein-cholesterol (HDL-C) is strongly correlated with presence of major occlusive vascular events.[9] Another key feature of diabetic lipophenotye is increased plasma triglyceride and reduced HDL-C level. In the Framingham Study, 19% of men and 17% of women with T2DM compared to only 9% of nondiabetic men and 8% of nondiabetic women had high triglyceride levels.[7] In the United Kingdom Prospective Diabetes Study, subjects with diabetes had 50% higher triglyceride levels than the general population.[10] The lipophenotype of type 1 diabetes is identical to that of T2DM with increased preponderance of dyslipidemia among females, high LDL-C, triglyceride, and low HDL-C levels.[11]

Asian Indians have a distinct lipophenotype that has some differences from Caucasian and other populations. While prevalence of raised LDL-C is not much different, hypertriglyceridemia and low HDL-C seem to be more common in Asian Indians. The ICMR-INDIAB study reported that 13.9% of diabetic individuals had hypercholesterolemia, 29.5% had hypertriglyceridemia, 72.3% had low HDL-C, 11.8% had high LDL-C levels, and 79% had abnormalities in at least one of the lipid parameters. The common risk factors for dyslipidemia included obesity, diabetes, and dysglycemia.[12] Moreover, despite similar BMI, Asian Indians have significantly greater total abdominal fat and visceral fat as compared to Caucasians, which predisposes them to an increased risk of dyslipidemia.[13]

ADIPOSE TISSUE DYSFUNCTION IN DIABETES

One of the key pathological defects that link obesity, metabolic syndrome, diabetes, and cardiovascular risk is a state of adipose tissue dysfunction. Several factors contribute to this including genetic predisposition, chronic over-nutrition with caloric excess and obesity, insulin resistance and the effect of endocrine disruptors or obesogens.

The underlying cause of altered adipocyte behavior in obesity remains poorly understood. Adipocyte injury (adipocyte tissue hypoxia) begins by decreased production of adiponectin and leptin. Reduced secretion of these mediators promote adipocyte lipolysis, inhibit mitochondrial energy production and activate the inhibitor κB kinase (IKK)/nuclear factor-κB (NF-κB) inflammatory pathway. The rapid expansion of adipocyte tissue leads to secretion of hypoxia-inducible factor-1α and vascular epithelial growth factor,[14,15] thus promoting angiogenesis, apoptosis, activation of macrophages, and marking the start of inflammation.

A characteristic lipid abnormality in diabetes is increased circulating FFAs. The FFA absorption from gut and their storage as triglycerides is regulated by serum insulin levels. Simultaneously, lipolysis in the adipocytes is inhibited under the effect of insulin. These pathways, along with reduced muscle and hepatic uptake lead to elevated FFA levels in diabetes.

Additionally, it has been proposed that proliferation of extracellular matrix, especially collagen type 4 and consequent adipose tissue fibrosis in T2DM and obesity limits adipocyte growth and causes metabolic dysregulation. The converse, absence of these fibrotic mechanisms and metabolic improvement have also been demonstrated.[16]

LIPOTOXICITY

Elevated FFAs can lead to significant insulin resistance, both in muscle and liver, and exacerbate impairment in insulin secretion, thus contributing to the key pathophysiological defects of diabetes. The effects of lipotoxicity on metabolic health seem to be mediated via several intracellular pathways, where it collaborates and is interlinked with the effects of chronic hyperglycemia/glucotoxicity and has effects on both short-term β-cell function and long-term β-cell survival and differentiation as well as insulin sensitivity. Some of these mechanisms include chronic inflammation, endoplasmic reticulum (ER) stress, oxidative stress, endothelial dysfunction and autophagy, and are discussed further.

Chronic overfeeding induced adipocyte hypertrophy with FFA excess leads to reduced proliferation and differentiation of the ER thereby triggering the unfolded protein response (UPR) as a protective mechanism. This is depicted in flowchart 1. The UPR consists of several adipocyte mediated inflammatory responses mediated via the c-Jun N-terminal kinase (c-JNK), IKK/NF-κB, and cyclic adenosine monophosphate-responsive element binding protein H (CREBH) signaling pathways. These responses further promote the secretion of acute phase reactants and reactive oxygen species (ROS).[17] Weight loss has shown benefit in reversing these disrupted pathways.[18]

Increased concentrations of FFAs, in the setting of obesity, inhibit insulin-stimulated activation of phosphatidylinositol 3-kinase (PI3K), protein kinase B (Akt), and vessel endothelial nitric oxide synthase leading to capillary and endothelial dysfunction.[19] This leads to macrophage activation, causing further adipocyte injury. Similar impairments have been documented in skeletal muscle in obese and

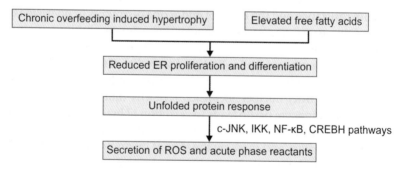

c-JNK, c-Jun N-terminal kinase; CREBH, cyclic AMP responsive element binding protein H; ER, endoplasmic reticulum; FFAs, free fatty acids; IKK, inhibitor κB kinase; NF-κB, nuclear factor κB; ROS, reactive oxygen species.

FLOWCHART 1: Chronic overfeeding and free fatty acid excess lead to increased reactive oxygen species and acute phase reactant protein secretion. Chronic overfeeding and increased FFA secretion from adipose tissue leads to endoplasmic reticulum stress and reduces ER proliferation and differentiation. This triggers UPR response which results in activation of several downstream inflammatory pathways including c-JNK, IKK, NF-κB and CREBH. These lead to increased oxidative stress and inflammation by increasing the secretion of ROS and acute phase reactant proteins.

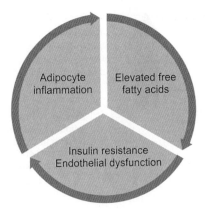

FIG. 1: The pathophysiological relationship between adipocyte dysfunction, elevated free fatty acid secretion, insulin resistance, and endothelial dysfunction.

T2DM subjects.[20] Figure 1 outlines the pathophysiological relationship between adipocyte dysfunction, elevated FFA secretion, insulin resistance, and endothelial dysfunction.

Other factors with possible role in lipotoxicity include direct stimulation of the proinflammatory NF-κB pathway by FFAs mediated via the toll-like receptor (TLR) family, especially TLR4, causing impaired insulin signaling and thus resistance; loss of regulation of lipid storage and trafficking in adipose tissue mediated by altered fatty acid–binding proteins; differential effect of various FFAs on monocyte adhesion and production of chemotactic factors; and role of CD95-mediated cellular apoptosis.[21]

LIPOTOXICITY AND INSULIN SECRETION

Free fatty acids can have both a positive and a negative effect on β-cell function, depending on the metabolic milieu, as depicted in figure 2. When FFA concentrations are in the physiological range, they help maintain glucose-stimulated insulin secretion (GSIS) through two key mechanisms:
- Effect on free fatty acid receptor 1 (FFAR-1): G-protein coupled receptor 40 (GPR40) or FFAR-1 is a G-protein coupled receptor expressed in islet cells. It acts as a nutrient sensor and regulates energy homeostasis. Activation of FFAR-1 leads to downstream activation of phospholipase C and hydrolysis of phosphatidyl-inositol-4,5-bisphosphate to diacylglycerol (DAG) and inositol triphosphate. Inositol triphosphate mediates an increase in cytosolic calcium influx to promote insulin secretion. Therefore, GPR40 agonists may have a potential role in diabetes management[22]
- Intracellular metabolism of FFA: Glucose and FFA metabolic pathways converge at the glycerolipid/FFA cycle that is primarily driven by substrates of glucose and FFA, glycerol-3-phosphate and fatty acyl-coenzyme A (CoA), respectively. At low concentrations of glucose such as during fasting, FFAs are the primary substrate for energy in islet cells. In the fed state, glucose increases the "switch" compound malonyl-CoA, that blocks mitochondrial β-oxidation of FFAs and increases fatty acyl-CoA, thereby causing a shift from fatty acid to glucose oxidation. This leads to

SECTION 2: Endocrine Aspects of Lipidology

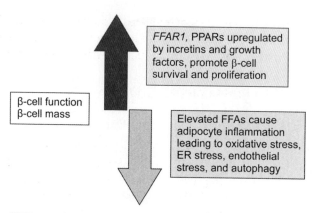

PPARs, peroxisome proliferator-activated receptors; FFAs, free fatty acids; FFAR-1, free fatty acid receptor-1; ER, endoplasmic reticulum.

FIG. 2: Effect of free fatty acids on pancreatic β-cells.

increased availability of fatty acyl-CoA for signaling pathways involved in insulin secretion.[22]

On the other hand, when the FFA concentrations are chronically elevated and in the presence of concomitant hyperglycemia, FFAs can have detrimental effects on insulin secretion, β-cell function and survival. Prolonged exposure of β-cells to long chain fatty acids such as palmitic acid leads to accumulation of potentially toxic lipids such as fatty acyl-CoA, DAG, ceramides, and others that act via several pathways to impair insulin secretion and increase β-cell apoptosis. Since β-cells can accommodate very limited quantity of triacylglycerol, it makes them susceptible to early FFA damage caused by accumulated toxic lipid metabolites (e.g., ceramide, DAG, and others). These lipid metabolites are diverted towards harmful metabolic pathways (palmitate esterification and lipolysis), leading to free radical damage and marked depletion of insulin stores.[23-25] *In vitro* and *in vivo* studies on animal models (Zucker diabetic fatty rats), have shown that chronic excess (24–48 h) of FFAs led to activation of the NF-κB pathway, formation of ROS, and lipid-induced β-cell apoptosis.[24] In addition, they also impair GSIS and insulin gene transcription and down regulate insulin receptor substrate 1/2 signaling. There is increased activation of protein kinase C-δ that mediates apoptosis. Cholesterol may also have some effect on β-cell health. Oxidized LDL has been shown to down regulate insulin gene transcription and promote β-cell apoptosis. Activation of ATP-binding cassette transporter A1 in human islets with liver X receptor agonists may improve GSIS.[22]

The lipotoxic injury to pancreatic β-cells is more pronounced in the presence of concomitant hyperglycemia as it leads to greater accumulation of long chain acyl-CoA esters in the cytosol, as in T2DM.[24] In nonobese normal glucose-tolerant subjects with a family history of diabetes, chronic lipid excess and infusion causes severe hepatic insulin resistance and reduced insulin secretion. Further reiterating this, it has been shown that treatment with acipimox, a nicotinic acid derivative that lowers plasma FFA levels, resulted in improved insulin secretion in subjects predisposed to T2DM.[26] Thus, mechanisms of both glucotoxicity and lipotoxicity may be vital in pathogenesis and development of T2DM.

Another important mechanism that regulates insulin secretion and β-cell survival is autophagy. The β-cells exposed to fatty acids accumulate abnormal autophagosome morphology and suppress lysosomal degradation, with impaired autophagic turnover.

LIPOTOXICITY: EFFECT ON INSULIN RESISTANCE

Hepatic Insulin Resistance and Fatty Liver Disease

The characteristic feature of T2DM, fasting hyperglycemia, is often linked with endogenous glucose production (EGP), which is regulated predominantly by the liver. Though the processes regulating glycogenolysis remain preserved until end stage disease, early increase of EGP in T2DM causes increased hepatic gluconeogenesis. There is evidence that mechanisms regulating these two pathways, along with insulin signaling are impaired by high plasma FFA concentrations. It has been demonstrated that in nonobese nondiabetic individuals, rapid lipid infusion leads to increase in plasma FFA and thus causes insulin resistance. Along with this, lipid mediated hepatic insulin resistance, adaptive mechanisms of body against insulin-resistance states reduce hepatic insulin clearance, resulting in hyperinsulinemia. This underlying lipotoxicity in the setting T2DM leads to hepatic tissue inflammation and injury through the intracellular mechanisms discussed above, thus causing nonalcoholic steatohepatitis and nonalcoholic fatty liver disease.[27]

Muscle Insulin Resistance

In trying to understand the role of obesity in the development of diabetes, it was seen that nonobese people with normal glucose tolerance and family history of diabetes, had insulin resistance before they developed impaired glucose tolerance, diabetes, or obesity.[26,28-30] This signifies that there is presence of an intrinsic genetic defect in the skeletal muscle of T2DM patients which precedes the onset of obesity or hyperglycemia. Studies in lean subjects with family history of T2DM have demonstrated that there is a significant impairment of insulin signaling from insulin receptor to PI3-K/IRS-1 to Akt and insulin-stimulated glycogen synthase fractional velocity.[28,29] This response remains unchanged when these subjects are exposed to elevated plasma FFA.[29] However, when lean insulin sensitive subjects with no family history are exposed to increasing plasma FFA concentrations, there is a rapid development of insulin resistance starting at plasma FFA concentrations within the range of 600–700 μmol/L. Hence, it can be concluded insulin-mediated skeletal muscle glucose uptake is very sensitive to excess lipid exposure.[31]

It has also been demonstrated that, excessive FFA availability leads to the accumulation of intramyocellular lipids (IMCLs) and the formation of fat-derived toxic lipid metabolites such as ceramide and DAG that cause insulin resistance. Muscle glucose oxidation is enhanced with training, a response blunted in the subjects with T2DM. Therefore, athletes despite having increased IMCLs, are extremely insulin sensitive, a paradox that is explained by their high muscle oxidative capacity. Hence, it can be inferred that insulin resistance is not caused by IMCL deposition, rather it is linked to reduced muscle lipid oxidation. It has been demonstrated in transgenic mice that overexpression of lipid oxidative enzymes leads to reduced DAG and ceramide content and is protective against lipotoxicity and insulin resistance. These mechanisms of mitochondrial oxidation capacity are reduced in lean individuals with family history of diabetes, and in patients with T2DM, indicating adverse role of underlying lipotoxicity. However, these mechanisms of FFA induced skeletal muscle insulin resistance remain controversial.[21]

ROLE OF PPARγ AND PGC1α IN LIPOTOXICITY

Peroxisome proliferator-activated receptor γ coactivator-1 α (PGC1α) has a vital role in regulating glucose homeostasis and fatty acid oxidation. It has been demonstrated that in obese subjects, severe restriction of calorie intake increases muscle PGC1α expression and reduces insulin resistance. Conversely, lipid excess, by infusion or high-fat diet, promotes alterations in mitochondrial oxidative phosphorylation activity and reduces PGC1α expression in skeletal muscle in as early as 3 days. These effects were not significant when studied on young healthy men. This discrepancy could be explained by errors in sample size and differences in intervention diet and duration.[32]

Similar actions have been described with activation of peroxisome proliferator-activated receptor γ (PPARγ) receptors. The PPARγ synthetic ligands, the glitazones, have been in use for treatment of T2DM for decades now. They improve insulin sensitivity, lower plasma blood glucose levels and reduce the rate of development of complications. They indirectly increase insulin-stimulated glucose uptake in adipocytes, hepatocytes, and skeletal muscle cells. These actions of PPARγ activation are partly caused by reduction in plasma FFA levels and increased adipocyte lipid storage, leading to reduced peripheral, skeletal muscle, and hepatic lipotoxicity. The commonly used PPARγ agonist pioglitazone increases HDL-C and decreases triglycerides and fasting plasma FFAs (without any influence on total cholesterol and LDL-C). Vascular endothelial dysfunction is also prevented by PPARγ activation along with reduction in blood pressure in patients with diabetes. Despite these numerous benefits, glitazones have some side effects which include, weight gain, edema, bone fractures, heart failure, and increased risk of myocardial infarction (the latter with rosiglitazone), which have limited the use of these drugs for management of dyslipidemia in T2DM.[33]

Another analogous class of drugs holding potential as treatment for lipotoxicity in T2DM is the PPARα/γ dual agonists. The PPARα acts by mediating lipid catabolism by β-oxidation, limiting inflammatory processes and maintaining endothelial function. Dual agonists ensure positive effects on both lipid and glucose metabolism. These may be effective treatment choices for managing dyslipidemia in T2DM; however, their abundant use is limited by side effects related to PPARγ agonistic activity, i.e., weight gain and edema. Most congeners of this drug class have been rejected for use in daily clinical practice because of the increased risk of bladder cancer and hyperplasia (ragaglitazar and naveglitazar)[34] or, renal dysfunction (tesaglitazar)[35] and increased cardiovascular risk (muraglitazar).[36] The only molecule which was approved for clinical use in India is saroglitazar, which effectively reduces triglycerides and non-HDL cholesterol and reduces insulin resistance. There have been no serious adverse events reported for this drug; however, long-term efficacy yet needs to be established.[37,38]

CONCLUSION

To sum up, though newer insights to understanding of cellular and molecular mechanisms of glucotoxicity and lipotoxicity in diabetes have been established, specific causal associations between cellular events and onset of diabetes are not thoroughly understood. Additional research is warranted to precisely elicit the effect of β-cell lipotoxicity in T2DM and identify relevant therapeutic targets for the same. Most research is limited due to complexity of developing an *in vivo* chronic over-nutrition study model, leading to use of *in vitro* models such as isolated islets or β-cell lines, which lack reliability and consistency. Also, the interplay of innumerable factors in development of these two chronic diseases, obesity and diabetes, make it very hard to mimic the *in vivo* human environment of disease development. Newer research methods, along with potential drug discovery targeting lipotoxicity mechanisms in the pathogenesis of diabetes may provide breakthrough development in effective management in future.

REFERENCES

1. DeFronzo RA. Insulin resistance, lipotoxicity, type 2 diabetes and atherosclerosis: The missing links. The Claude Bernard Lecture 2009. Diabetologia. 2010;53(7):1270-87.
2. Unnikrishnan R, Anjana RM, Mohan V. Diabetes mellitus and its complications in India. Nat Rev Endocrinol. 2016;12(6):357-70.
3. Pradeepa R, Anjana RM, Joshi SR, et al. Prevalence of generalized & abdominal obesity in urban & rural India--the ICMR-INDIAB Study (Phase-I) [ICMR- NDIAB-3]. Indian J Med Res. 2015;142(2):139-50.
4. Ranjani H, Mehreen TS, Pradeepa R, et al. Epidemiology of childhood overweight & obesity in India: A systematic review. Indian J Med Res. 2016;143(2):160-74.
5. Raj M. Obesity and cardiovascular risk in children and adolescents. Indian J Endocrinol Metab. 2012;16(1):13-9.
6. Franks PW, Hanson RL, Knowler WC, et al. Childhood obesity, other cardiovascular risk factors, and premature death. N Engl J Med. 2010;362(6):485-93.
7. Kannel WB. Lipids, diabetes, and coronary heart disease: Insights from the Framingham Study. Am Heart J. 1985;110(5):1100-7.
8. Jacobs MJ, Kleisli T, Pio JR, et al. Prevalence and control of dyslipidemia among persons with diabetes in the United States. Diabetes Res Clin Pract. 2005;70(3):263-9.
9. Parish S, Offer A, Clarke R, et al. Lipids and lipoproteins and risk of different vascular events in the MRC/BHF Heart Protection Study. Circulation. 2012;125(20):2469-78.
10. U.K. Prospective Diabetes Study 27. Plasma lipids and lipoproteins at diagnosis of NIDDM by age and sex. Diabetes Care. 1997;20(11):1683-7.
11. Marcovecchio ML, Dalton RN, Prevost AT, et al. Prevalence of abnormal lipid profiles and the relationship with the development of microalbuminuria in adolescents with type 1 diabetes. Diabetes Care. 2009;32(4):658-63.
12. Joshi SR, Anjana RM, Deepa M, et al. Prevalence of dyslipidemia in urban and rural India: The ICMR-INDIAB study. PLoS One. 2014;9(5):e96808.
13. Raji A, Seely EW, Arky RA, et al. Body fat distribution and insulin resistance in healthy Asian Indians and Caucasians. J Clin Endocrinol Metab. 2001;86(11):5366-71.
14. Rutkowski JM, Davis KE, Scherer PE. Mechanisms of obesity and related pathologies: The macro- and microcirculation of adipose tissue. FEBS J. 2009;276(20):5738-46.
15. Ye J. Emerging role of adipose tissue hypoxia in obesity and insulin resistance. Int J Obes (Lond). 2009;33(1):54-66.
16. Khan T, Muise ES, Iyengar P, et al. Metabolic dysregulation and adipose tissue fibrosis: Role of collagen VI. Mol Cell Biol. 2009;29(6):1575-91.

SECTION 2: Endocrine Aspects of Lipidology

17. Hotamisligil GS, Erbay E. Nutrient sensing and inflammation in metabolic diseases. Nat Rev Immunol. 2008;8(12):923-34.
18. Gregor MF, Yang L, Fabbrini E, et al. Endoplasmic reticulum stress is reduced in tissues of obese subjects after weight loss. Diabetes. 2009;58(3):693-700.
19. Muniyappa R, Iantorno M, Quon MJ. An integrated view of insulin resistance and endothelial dysfunction. Endocrinol Metab Clin North Am. 2008;37(3):685-711.
20. Cusi K, Maezono K, Osman A, et al. Insulin resistance differentially affects the PI 3-kinase- and MAP kinase-mediated signaling in human muscle. J Clin Invest. 2000;105(3):311-20.
21. Cusi K. The role of adipose tissue and lipotoxicity in the pathogenesis of type 2 diabetes. Curr Diab Rep. 2010;10(4):306-15.
22. Sharma RB, Alonso LC. Lipotoxicity in the pancreatic beta cell: Not just survival and function, but proliferation as well? Curr Diab Rep. 2014;14(6):492.
23. Delghingaro-Augusto V, Nolan CJ, Gupta D, et al. Islet beta cell failure in the 60% pancreatectomised obese hyperlipidaemic Zucker fatty rat: Severe dysfunction with altered glycerolipid metabolism without steatosis or a falling beta cell mass. Diabetologia. 2009;52(6):1122-32.
24. Poitout V, Robertson RP. Glucolipotoxicity: Fuel excess and beta-cell dysfunction. Endocr Rev. 2008;29(3):351-66.
25. Unger RH, Zhou YT. Lipotoxicity of beta-cells in obesity and in other causes of fatty acid spillover. Diabetes. 2001;50(Suppl 1):S118-21.
26. Kashyap S, Belfort R, Gastaldelli A, et al. A sustained increase in plasma free fatty acids impairs insulin secretion in nondiabetic subjects genetically predisposed to develop type 2 diabetes. Diabetes. 2003;52(10):2461-74.
27. Zambo V, Simon-Szabo L, Szelenyi P, et al. Lipotoxicity in the liver. World J Hepatol. 2013;5(10):550-7.
28. Pratipanawatr W, Pratipanawatr T, Cusi K, et al. Skeletal muscle insulin resistance in normoglycemic subjects with a strong family history of type 2 diabetes is associated with decreased insulin-stimulated insulin receptor substrate-1 tyrosine phosphorylation. Diabetes. 2001;50(11):2572-8.
29. Kashyap SR, Belfort R, Berria R, et al. Discordant effects of a chronic physiological increase in plasma FFA on insulin signaling in healthy subjects with or without a family history of type 2 diabetes. Am J Physiol Endocrinol Metab. 2004;287(3):E537-46.
30. Gulli G, Ferrannini E, Stern M, et al. The metabolic profile of NIDDM is fully established in glucose-tolerant offspring of two Mexican-American NIDDM parents. Diabetes. 1992;41(12):1575-86.
31. Belfort R, Mandarino L, Kashyap S, et al. Dose-response effect of elevated plasma free fatty acid on insulin signaling. Diabetes. 2005;54(6):1640-8.
32. Puigserver P, Spiegelman BM. Peroxisome proliferator-activated receptor-gamma coactivator 1 alpha (PGC-1 alpha): Transcriptional coactivator and metabolic regulator. Endocr Rev. 2003;24(1):78-90.
33. Monsalve FA, Pyarasani RD, Delgado-Lopez F, et al. Peroxisome proliferator-activated receptor targets for the treatment of metabolic diseases. Mediators Inflamm. 2013;2013:549627.
34. Long GG, Reynolds VL, Lopez-Martinez A, et al. Urothelial carcinogenesis in the urinary bladder of rats treated with naveglitazar, a gamma-dominant PPAR alpha/gamma agonist: lack of evidence for urolithiasis as an inciting event. Toxicol Pathol. 2008;36(2):218-31.
35. Wilding JP, Gause-Nilsson I, Persson A. Tesaglitazar, as add-on therapy to sulphonylurea, dose-dependently improves glucose and lipid abnormalities in patients with type 2 diabetes. Diab Vasc Dis Res. 2007;4(3):194-203.
36. Nissen SE, Wolski K, Topol EJ. Effect of muraglitazar on death and major adverse cardiovascular events in patients with type 2 diabetes mellitus. JAMA. 2005;294(20):2581-6.
37. Munigoti SP, Harinarayan CV. Role of glitazars in atherogenic dyslipidemia and diabetes: Two birds with one stone? Indian J Endocrinol Metab. 2014;18(3):283-7.
38. Shetty SR, Kumar S, Mathur RP, et al. Observational study to evaluate the safety and efficacy of saroglitazar in Indian diabetic dyslipidemia patients. Indian Heart J. 2015;67(1):23-6.

CHAPTER 10

The Asian Lipophenotype

Altamash Shaikh

> **ABSTRACT**
>
> There are quantitative and qualitative differences in health and disease between Asians and non-Asians. Asian phenotype is clearly distinct from the rest, making them more prone for certain diseases especially diabetes, metabolic syndrome, and heart disease. The atherogenic dyslipidemia that Asians manifest, called as Asian lipophenotype, has its own characteristic properties. Differences between Asians and non-Asians in the lipophenotype are discussed in the light of anatomic, anthropometric, epidemiologic, therapeutic, and genetic implications. Differences in prevalence, morbidity, and mortality and response to lipid-lowering drugs are also discussed.

INTRODUCTION

Who are Asians? Around 60% of the current mankind, the native inhabitants of the largest continent of Asia, are termed Asians. Here in this chapter, "Asian phenotype" would mean individuals of Asian origin who possess a distinct anthropometric and metabolic phenotype as elaborated subsequently. Synonyms of Asian phenotype include "South Asian" or "South East Asian phenotype" or "Asian Indian phenotype." Asians also differ from other ethnic groups in their phenotypic characteristics in relation to several other diseases such as thyrotoxic periodic paralysis, Brugada syndrome, nasopharyngeal carcinoma, etc. Before we proceed further in the chapter, it is vital to first delineate the differences between Asians and non-Asians.

WHY DIFFERENTIATE: NON-ASIAN VERSUS ASIAN?

Not only in genotype but also in phenotype, there are differences between Asians and non-Asians which bears implications in health and disease. Asians have (i) smaller body size, (ii) more truncal and abdominal adiposity, (iii) lower average waist circumference, and (iv) higher waist/hip circumference ratio as compared to non-Asians of similar body mass index (BMI).[1] Thus, there is a distinct "thin outside

TABLE 1: Phenotypic differences between Asians and non-Asians

Parameters	Asian	Non-Asian
Body frame	Smaller	Larger
Birth weight	Lower	Higher
Fat pockets at any BMI	More truncal, abdominal	Less
Adipocytes	Large, dysfunctional	Smaller, functional
Fat percentage at same BMI	3–5% higher	Lower
Frank obesity	Lower	Higher
Adiponectin	Lower	Higher
Insulin resistance, any BMI	More	Lesser
Insulin sensitivity	Less	More
Glycemic response	Higher	Much less
Muscle volume	Less	More
Waist circumference	Lower	More
Waist/hip ratio	Higher	Lower
Overall phenotype	Thin outside fat inside	Thin outside muscle inside

BMI, body mass index.

TABLE 2: Waist circumference in Asians and non-Asians

Waist circumference	NCEP ATP III (USA)	IDF (Europid)	IDF (Asians)
Men (cm)	>102	>94	>90
Women (cm)	>88	80	>80

NCEP ATP III, National Cholesterol Education Program Adult Treatment Panel III; IDF, International Diabetes Federation.

fat inside" characteristic phenotype that predisposes to visceral obesity and type 2 diabetes mellitus (T2DM) at relatively lower BMI. This is also termed as the South Asian or Asian Indian phenotype. Table 1 delineates these differences in anatomic, anthropometric, histological and metabolic features between Asians and non-Asians/Caucasians.

A higher prevalence of abdominal and visceral adiposity in Asians compared to other ethnicities led to recognition of lower cutoffs to define obesity in Asians than was originally proposed in the diagnostic guidelines for metabolic syndrome, the National Cholesterol Education Program Adult Treatment Panel III.[2] The cut-offs for waist circumference to define obesity in men and women of Asian and non-Asian origin are described in table 2.[3] These phenotypic characteristics are associated with a higher prevalence of T2DM, dyslipidemia, hypertension, metabolic syndrome, and cardiovascular disease (CVD), as has been documented in urban and migrant Asian Indian populations.

THE "ASIAN LIPOPHENOTYPE": ATHEROGENIC DYSLIPIDEMIA

The combination of dysglycemia with specific dyslipidemias is a hallmark of South Asian phenotype. At levels of overall body mass considered normal in other

populations, Asians manifest greater prevalence of lipid alterations and dyslipidemias and this can be described as Asian lipophenotype.[4] The pattern of lipid abnormalities includes:
- Reduced high-density lipoprotein cholesterol (HDL-C), with shift towards smaller dysfunctional HDL particles
- Elevated triglycerides and very low-density lipoprotein (VLDL)
- Elevated low-density lipoprotein cholesterol (LDL-C), especially small dense LDL
- Elevated triglycerides related to HDL-C
- Elevated lipoprotein(a).

The mechanisms leading to these lipid alterations in Asians and their role in CVD are discussed subsequently.

FACTORS CONTRIBUTING TO THE ASIAN PHENOTYPE

The phenotypic characteristics that distinguish Asians from other ethnicities have been attributed to result from a multitude of factors including genetic as well as environmental. Individuals from different continents have approximately 9–13% genetic variation that may affect the phenotype. Asians have a genetic predisposition to dyslipidemia and CVD as has been demonstrated in several genome-wide association studies (GWAS) discussed later. Other factors include environmental stressors and triggers, nutritional transition, sedentary lifestyle, population migration, and urbanization.[5] In addition, maternal and fetal malnutrition, low birth weight and poor intrauterine and early life growth have been proposed to predispose to greater risk of metabolic abnormalities as adults.[6,7] Indeed, evaluation of intrauterine growth and body composition of Asian Indian babies has demonstrated a tendency to preservation of adiposity and paucity of muscle mass in them.[6]

Several hypotheses have been forwarded to explain the rapid increase in diabetes, CVD, and associated metabolic abnormalities in certain populations and include:
- Thrifty genotype—conservation of energy-conserving thrifty genes which are advantageous in periods of nutritional deprivation but detrimental in an environment of nutrient surplus[5]
- Thrifty phenotype—reduced intrauterine growth predisposes to obesity and metabolic disorders in later life. Poor intrauterine environment and limited nutrient supply may result in metabolic adaptive changes in fetus, that turn out to be detrimental later. This has also been described as the fetal origins hypothesis.[5]

In addition to thrifty genotype and phenotype, gestational diabetes, intergenerational issues, and masking of silent genes may also be responsible for the Asian phenotype. Also, there is a different ancestry-specific human phenotype, as confirmed by GWAS, in the "Asian phenotype" for T2DM.

CORONARY ARTERY DISEASE IN ASIANS

Coronary artery disease (CAD) prevalence rates in the last few decades showed an increase from 2% in 1970 to 4.5% in 2000 in the rural areas and from 2% in 1960 to 10.5% in 2000 in the urban areas.[8] An Asian Indian individual's risk of CAD is nearly 4, 6, and 20 times higher than Caucasians, Chinese, and Japanese, respectively.[8]

Whereas CAD related deaths in people below the age of 70 years was only 22% in developed countries, they were 52% in India.[9] The age-standardized CAD mortality analysis in Canada over a 15-year period has revealed that South Asians including people from India, Pakistan, Sri Lanka, Nepal, and Bangladesh have a higher mortality as compared to people of Chinese and European descent.[10]

HOW COMMON IS DYSLIPIDEMIA AMONG ASIANS?

Combined dyslipidemia and elevated LDL-C are traditionally associated with a significantly increased risk of CVD. However, hypertriglyceridemia and low HDL-C also contribute to CV risk and this is particularly important for Asians.

Large studies like National Health and Nutrition Examination Survey (NHANES) (United States) have shown that 47% of the population had triglyceride levels of more than 150 mg/dL and these increased levels were driven mainly by lifestyle factors.[11] Data from the European continent also suggests that 27% of all adults have a nonfasting triglyceride level of more than 2.0 mmol/L (>176 mg/dL).[11] A systematic review of 16 studies, comprising of 32,905 individuals from countries of South Asia, found the prevalence of hypertriglyceridemia to be 37.2%, with majority of these studies (n = 10) having been conducted in India. Of these 16 studies, 13 studies reported a prevalence of hypertriglyceridemia in the range varying from 25.2 to 55.1%.[12] In India, there are only a few population-based studies on cholesterol and other lipoprotein lipid levels.[13]

Of the few large studies, the India Heart Watch study (n = 6,123) conducted among urban middle class subjects in 11 cities of India, reported a prevalence of hypertriglyceridemia of 42.1% in men and 32.9% in women.[14] The first phase of the ICMR INDIAB (Indian Council of Medical Research–India Diabetes) study (n = 2,042), which was restricted to urban and rural populations in four states of India, reported hypertriglyceridemia as the second most common dyslipidemia at 29.5% of the population after low HDL-C which was seen in 72.3%.[13] Another large study of 67,000 participants using a fasting sample and sourced from the hospital administrative database, found the prevalence of hypertriglyceridemia to be 34% in men and 26.8% in women, respectively.[15] The pan-India, industry driven, FitHeart study (n = 46,919) conducted in more than 20 states of India utilized a camp approach and found the prevalence of hypertriglyceridemia to be 42.6% (men 45.6%, women 38.6%).[15] The lack of additional large population-based studies with a detailed pattern of dyslipidemia, in India has been a major drawback. Overall, when compared to Western populations, Indians and migrant South Asians tend to have higher triglycerides values and lower HDL-C levels with total cholesterol being lower than their Western counterparts.[16]

ROLE OF ASIAN LIPOPHENOTYPE IN CARDIOVASCULAR DISEASE RISK

The importance of HDL-C levels in relation to CVD has long been debated and recent studies imply that rather than low levels of HDL-C, it is the disturbed functionality of HDL particles that contributes to atherosclerotic disease. The combined occurrence of hypertriglyceridemia and reduced HDL-C has been found to be metabolically interlinked and has been named as atherogenic dyslipidemia.[17] Atherogenic dyslipidemia is strongly associated with insulin resistance, increased levels of circulating free fatty acids, triglyceride-rich lipoproteins and small dense LDL-C particles, and is particularly common in south Asians. Atherogenic dyslipidemia has a strong corelation with T2DM, metabolic syndrome, and coronary heart disease (CHD).

Epidemiological evidence helps us in understanding the biological variations in health and the pathophysiological mechanisms of disease. Since the 1980s, several epidemiological studies have shown that triglycerides play an important role as an independent CV risk factor. In the PROVE IT-TIMI 22 (Pravastatin or Atorvastatin Evaluation and Infection Therapy–Thrombolysis in Myocardial Infarction 22) trial, it was observed that in individuals on statin therapy after an acute coronary syndrome, an on-treatment fasting triglyceride level of 150 mg/dL was linked with a decrease in recurrent coronary heart disease risk as compared to higher triglyceride levels, and this risk was present even on adjustment for HDL-C and LDL-C levels (HR 0.8; $p = 0.025$).[18]

In multiple studies, after correction for other risk factors like smoking, hypertension, BMI, diabetes, and blood glucose, even a slight elevation of triglyceride levels is linked with an increased risk of recurrent CVD in patients treated with statins and it can be considered as a useful marker of residual risk.[19] Triglycerides are an independent marker of increased risk for CV events even in patients who have attained recommended goals for LDL-C.

In a Japanese study of 30,378 patients who were followed up for 15 years, particularly in patients with low LDL-C levels, it was observed that elevated triglyceride levels predicted CAD, highlighting the fact that in patients with low LDL-C levels, other lipid fractions need to be considered for active management.[20] In a large Korean cohort of 86,476 individuals who had undergone a general health check-up between 2007 and 2011 and their data sourced for CVD events and death, it was observed that elevated triglyceride levels were independently associated with an increased risk of major CVD events [odds ratio (OR) 1.52, 95% confidence interval (CI) 1.27–1.82], major ischemic heart disease events (OR 1.53, 95% CI 1.24–1.88), and overall CVD events (OR 1.49, 95% CI 1.37–1.63). These risk estimates prevailed despite adjustment for multiple risk factors including HDL-C levels. This further highlights the significance of lipid alterations in Asian subjects and their relationship with CV risk.[21]

In a recent publication, higher triglyceride levels were found to be independently associated with an increased 22-year all-cause mortality in more than 15,000 patients. The 22-year risk of death in patients with triglyceride levels more than or equal to 500 mg/dL was significantly increased by 68% ($p < 0.001$) and in those with moderate hypertriglyceridemia (triglyceride levels 200–499 mg/dL), it was increased by 29% ($p < 0.001$) when compared to patients who had low normal triglyceride levels.[22]

The Strong Heart Study, recently published in 2017, was a prospective cohort of 3,216 American Indians who were free from CVD at baseline and were followed up for a period of 17.7 years. It was observed in this study that those participants who had high triglycerides (≥150 mg/dL) and low HDL-C levels (≤40 mg/dL for men, ≤50 for women) had a 32% higher risk for CHD as compared to those with normal triglycerides and normal HDL-C levels. Among diabetics, high triglyceride and low HDL-C levels were associated with a significant 54% greater risk for CHD (p = 0.003) and 2.13-fold greater risk for stroke (p = 0.060).[23]

Therefore, it is obvious that the Asian lipophenotype is associated with a significantly higher risk for cardiovascular morbidity and mortality. This is evident even in those who do not manifest the classic phenotype of atherogenic dyslipidemia but have subtle abnormalities in lipid parameters.

GENOTYPE ASSOCIATIONS WITH CARDIOVASCULAR RISK

Several gene polymorphisms have been implicated in the pathogenesis of CAD in the Asian population.[24] Table 3 enlists some of the reported genotypes that determine the risk of CAD in Asian Indians. However, presently, there is limited information on the reported genetic factors contributing to Asian lipophenotype and CAD in Asians.

In a meta-analysis of 188,578 genotyped individuals with 185 diverse single nucleotide polymorphisms, it was observed that the strength of a variant's effect on triglyceride levels matched with the extent of its effect on CAD, which was seen even after adjustments for LDL-C and HDL-C.[25]

A recent study, which screened 18,666 genes in 3,734 participants, identified four loss of function mutations in *APOC3*, the gene that encodes apolipoprotein C-III (apoC-III). Forty-six percent lower levels of circulating apoC-III were observed in the heterozygous carriers, which corresponded to 39% lower levels of triglycerides, and a 40% lesser risk of CHD as compared to the non-carriers.[26]

Mutations in the genes encoding apoA-V (APOA5), which activates lipoprotein lipase, are linked with CVD risk. These carriers had a 2.2-fold higher risk of myocardial infarction and CAD as compared to the non-carriers.[27]

TABLE 3 Reported coronary artery disease genotype in Asians

Genes	Associated Asian lipophenotype-related traits
ABCA1	Premature CAD, plasma levels of HDL-C, triglycerides and cholesterol
LIPH	CAD, plasma levels of triglyceride and HDL
CETP	CVD, CETP activity, plasma levels of triglycerides and HDL
APOE	Premature CAD and MI, hypertension, stroke, dyslipidemia and accelerated atherosclerosis, plasma levels of triglycerides and lipoprotein(a), serum apoE levels
APOA1	CAD, plasma lipid and apoA-I levels
APOA5	Premature CAD, serum triglycerides, pancreatitis, diabetes
APOC3	CAD, hypertension, plasma triglycerides, TC, HDL-C and apoB levels
LPA	CVD, obesity, carotid stenosis, serum homocysteine, uric acid, plasma lipoprotein(a) and CRP levels
LPL	Serum HDL-C and triglyceride levels

CAD, coronary artery disease; HDL-C, high-density lipoprotein cholesterol; CETP, cholesteryl ester transfer protein; TC, total cholesterol; CVD, cardiovascular disease.

MANAGEMENT CONSIDERATIONS IN DYSLIPIDEMIA AMONG ASIANS

Although primary trial data with lipid-lowering drugs for Asian population is sparse and largely extrapolated from studies based on a predominant Western population, there are several management considerations unique to the Asian lipophenotype. The pertinent issues relate to lifestyle intervention, threshold for the initiation of lipid-lowering treatment, choice, efficacy and tolerability of hypolipidemic drugs, and lipid targets among Asians.

Asians differ from people of non-Asian origin in not only their genetic make-up, but also in their sociocultural background. Eating behaviors and lifestyle patterns differ widely across regions and ethnicities and influence the manifestation and prognosis of chronic metabolic diseases. Therefore, it is important to develop culturally sensitive and individually tailored treatment plans, that includes both lifestyle intervention and pharmacological management.

There is a general trend towards rise in total cholesterol in Indian subjects as reported in some studies and there is a consistent pattern of high triglycerides and low HDL-C.[28]

The Lipid Association of India, in 2017, provides the most recent India-specific guidelines for the management of dyslipidemia in Asian Indians.[28] The major risk factors for atherosclerotic cardiovascular disease (ASCVD) include:

- Age 45 years and above in men and 55 years and above in women
- Family history of premature CAD or CVD in a first degree relative (<55 years in men and <65 years in women)
- Current cigarette smoking or tobacco chewing
- High blood pressure
- Low HDL-C (<40 mg/dL in men and <50 mg/dL in women).

Other features such as diabetes, chronic kidney disease, coronary artery calcium score, lipoprotein(a) levels may also be useful in risk assessment. This is outlined in flowchart 1 derived from the Lipid Association guidelines of India, 2017.[28] Lipoprotein(a) more than 20 mg/dL can be considered as an important marker for the risk of ASCVD in Indians, but its routine use is not yet recommended. The JBS3 (Joint British Society) risk calculator has been recommended as the most inclusive in Indian patients for estimation of CV risk.[28]

In recent times, there has been a nutritional shift with increased consumption of calorie-dense foods rich in refined carbohydrates and saturated fat, and concomitant decrease in the intake of proteins, fiber, and vegetables. This is accompanied by significantly reduced levels of physical activity, chronic stress and increased smoking. Therefore, it is important to emphasize on the need for dietary modification with reduced intake of saturated fats and increasing physical activity. Yoga and stress management may also be useful adjuncts to treatment.

While LDL-C remains the primary target, most international guidelines recommend non-HDL cholesterol as a preferred risk indicator and secondary target, particularly in patients with insulin resistance and elevated triglycerides.[29] Non-HDL cholesterol is simply the total cholesterol present in LDL, intermediate density lipoprotein, and VLDL particles, where VLDL is the main carrier of triglycerides. The Lipid Association of India consensus recommends non-HDL

SECTION 2: Endocrine Aspects of Lipidology

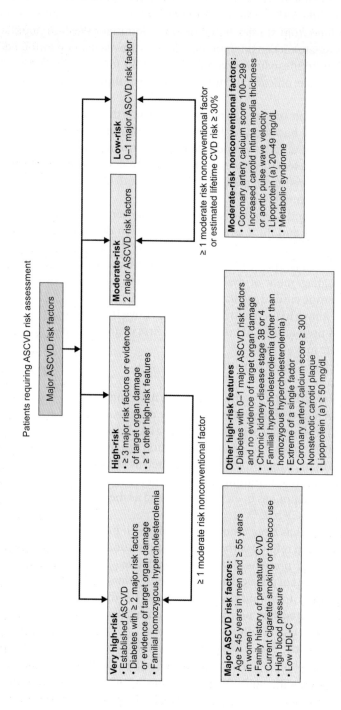

ASCVD, atherosclerotic cardiovascular disease; CVD, cardiovascular disease; HDL-C, high-density lipoprotein cholesterol.

FLOWCHART 1: Recommended approach to atherosclerotic cardiovascular disease risk stratification.

TABLE 4 Threshold for initiation of statins and therapeutic goals according to atherosclerotic cardiovascular disease risk category

Risk category	Consider initiation of drug therapy		Treatment goal	
	LDL-C (mg/dL)	Non-HDL-C (mg/dL)	LDL-C (mg/dL)	Non-HDL-C (mg/dL)
Very high-risk	≥50	≥80	<50	<80
High-risk	≥70	≥100	<70	<100
Moderate-risk	≥100	≥130	<100	<130
Low-risk	≥130	≥160	<100	<130

LDL-C, low-density lipoprotein cholesterol; HDL-C, high-density lipoprotein cholesterol.
Adapted from: TG and HDL Working Group of the Exome Sequencing Project, National Heart, Lung, and Blood Institute, Crosby J, Peloso GM, Auer PL, et al. Loss-of-function mutations in APOC3, triglycerides, and coronary disease. N Engl J Med. 2014;371(1):22-31.

cholesterol as a coprimary target, as important as LDL-C, for decision-making in initiation and monitoring of lipid-lowering drugs to reduce the ASCVD risk.[28] Non-HDL cholesterol is especially useful in those with hypertriglyceridemia and those already taking statins. Table 4 provides the recommendations for initiation of statins and treatment thresholds as per the Lipid Association of India guidelines.

Differences may also exist in drug metabolism between different races and ethnicities, leading to differences in the efficacy and safety of specific drugs. Statins remain the first line drugs for lipid-lowering in Asian Indians. The maximum approved dose for rosuvastatin is lower for Asians (includes South Asians) compared with others.[30] The initial rosuvastatin recommended dose is 5 mg once daily and maximum recommended dose 20 mg daily for Asians.[28,31] In studies comparing rosuvastatin and atorvastatin in Asian Indians, rosuvastatin was found to have better efficacy.[28,31,32] It has been observed that relatively lower statin doses may have a similar therapeutic effect in individuals of Asian origin compared to higher doses in other ethnic groups. This may be explained by genetic differences in statin metabolism, but overall data from various trials has yielded mixed results. Most recently, the CURE-ACS (Clopidogrel in Unstable Angina to Prevent Recurrent Events-Acute Coronary Syndromes) trial from India demonstrated that atorvastatin 80 mg daily was more effective than 40 mg in LDL reduction, and such high dose statin therapy was well-tolerated in these subjects who had a recent acute coronary syndrome.[33]

Other lipid-lowering drugs including fibrates, ezetimibe, saroglitazar, and others have also been recommended in Indian population when different components of dyslipidemia are not at goal. They may be considered if non-HDL cholesterol targets are not being achieved with the maximally tolerated dose of statins. For individuals with hypertriglyceridemia, it is important to exclude secondary causes of dyslipidemia such as uncontrolled diabetes or hypothyroidism, and intensive lifestyle modification should be implemented. Routine use of fibrates for lowering of triglycerides is not recommended, unless triglycerides are more than 500 mg/dL.[28] Fibrates may be considered if triglycerides are not sufficiently lowered with lifestyle modification and statins. Lifestyle modification and statins remain the primary options for raising HDL-C, as there is no evidence that HDL raising drugs offer clinical benefits.

BOX 1	Implications of Asian lipophenotype
<ul><li>More cardiovascular disease morbidity and mortality</li><li>Atherogenic dyslipidemia</li><li>Epidemiologists</li><li>Geneticists</li><li>Pharmaceuticals</li></ul>	<ul><li>Pharmacogenomics</li><li>Health and disease, daily clinical practice outcomes</li><li>Anthropometrics and anatomists</li><li>Global matter of further research: Beyond lipids</li></ul>

FUTURE CONSIDERATIONS

The interindividual variations of such magnitude that define the Asian phenotype and lipophenotype have major impact in health, disease and long-term outcomes. The understanding of these distinct phenotypic characteristics also opens a pandora of possibilities for the primary care physicians, endocrinologists, cardiologists, lipidologists, and nutritionists in their day to day clinical practice. This is further outlined in box 1. In addition, it holds profound significance for pharmaceutical research to identify drugs, drug combinations and tailor-made therapies that would reduce the global burden of CVD.

CONCLUSION

The Asian phenotype defines the anthropometric and metabolic features unique to individuals of Asian descent that has implications in health as well as disease. These phenotypic differences in metabolic and cardiovascular health have a bearing on the risk of chronic disorders including obesity, metabolic syndrome, diabetes, hypertension, dyslipidemia, and CVD. The lipid alterations in Asians that contribute to an increased cardiovascular risk include reduced HDL-C, raised triglycerides, small dense LDL-C, and elevated lipoprotein(a). An understanding of these differences is important for several health-related disciplines and holds significance for epidemiologists, geneticists, physicians, pharmaceuticals, and researchers globally. Culturally tailored prevention and intervention should be provided to various populations with dyslipidemia.

REFERENCES

1. Misra A, Vikram NK. Insulin resistance syndrome (metabolic syndrome) and obesity in Asian Indians: Evidence and implications. Nutrition. 2004;20(5):482-91.
2. National Cholesterol Education Program (NCEP) Expert Panel on Detection, Evaluation, and Treatment of High Blood Cholesterol in Adults (Adult Treatment Panel III). Third Report of the National Cholesterol Education Program (NCEP) Expert Panel on Detection, Evaluation, and Treatment of High Blood Cholesterol in Adults (Adult Treatment Panel III) final report. Circulation. 2002;106(25):3143-421.
3. Misra A, Chowbey P, Makkar BM, et al. Concensus Group. Consensus statement for diagnosis of obesity, abdominal obesity and the metabolic syndrome for Asian Indians and recommendations for physical activity, medical and surgical management. J Assoc Physicians India. 2009;57:163-70.
4. Enas EA, Mohan V, Deepa M, et al. The metabolic syndrome and dyslipidemia among Asian Indians: A population with high rates of diabetes and premature coronary artery disease. J Cardiometab Syndr. 2007 Fall;2(4):267-75.

5. Yajnik CS. Obesity epidemic in India: intrauterine origins? Proc Nutr Soc. 2004;63(3):387-96.
6. Sachdev HS, Fall CH, Osmond C, et al. Anthropometric indicators of body composition in young adults: relation to size at birth and serial measurements of body mass index in childhood in the New Delhi birth cohort. Am J Clin Nutr. 2005;82(2):456-66.
7. Fall CH, Sachdev HS, Osmond C, et al. New Delhi Birth Cohort. Adult metabolic syndrome and impaired glucose tolerance are associated with different patterns of BMI gain during infancy: Data from the New Delhi Birth Cohort. Diabetes Care. 2008;31(12):2349-56.
8. Gupta R. Recent trends in coronary heart disease epidemiology in India. Indian Heart J. 2008;60(2 Suppl B):B4-18.
9. Bahl VK, Prabhakaran D, Karthikeyan G. Coronary artery disease in Indians. Indian Heart J. 2001;53(6):707-13.
10. Sheth T, Nair C, Nargundkar M, et al. Cardiovascular and cancer mortality among Canadians of European, south Asian and Chinese origin from 1979 to 1993: An analysis of 1.2 million deaths. CMAJ. 1999;161(2):132-8.
11. Nordestgaard BG. Triglyceride-rich lipoproteins and atherosclerotic cardiovascular disease: New insights from epidemiology, genetics, and biology. Circ Res. 2016;118(4):547-63.
12. Aryal N, Wasti SP. The prevalence of metabolic syndrome in South Asia: A systematic review. Int J Diabetes Dev Ctries. 2016;36(3):255-62.
13. Gupta R, Guptha S, Sharma KK, et al. Regional variations in cardiovascular risk factors in India: India heart watch. World J Cardiol. 2012;4(4):112-20.
14. Gupta R, Sharma M, Goyal NK, et al. Gender differences in 7 years trends in cholesterol lipoproteins and lipids in India: Insights from a hospital database. Indian J Endocrinol Metab. 2016;20(2):211-8.
15. Chandra KS, Bansal M, Nair T, et al. Consensus statement on management of dyslipidemia in Indian subjects. Indian Heart J. 2014;66 Suppl 3:S1-51.
16. Enas EA, Dharmarajan TS, Varkey B. Consensus statement on the management of dyslipidemia in Indian subjects: A different perspective. Indian Heart J. 2015;67(2):95-102.
17. Misra A, Shrivastava U. Obesity and dyslipidemia in South Asians. Nutrients. 2013;5(7):2708-33.
18. Miller M, Cannon CP, Murphy SA, et al.; PROVE IT-TIMI 22 Investigators. Impact of triglyceride levels beyond low-density lipoprotein cholesterol after acute coronary syndrome in the PROVE IT-TIMI 22 trial. J Am Coll Cardiol. 2008;51(7):724-30.
19. Emerging Risk Factors Collaboration, Di Angelantonio E, Sarwar N, Perry P, et al. Major lipids, apolipoproteins, and risk of vascular disease. JAMA. 2009;302(18):1993-2000.
20. Iso H, Imano H, Yamagishi K, et al. CIRCS Investigators. Fasting and non-fasting triglycerides and risk of ischemic cardiovascular disease in Japanese men and women: The Circulatory Risk in Communities Study (CIRCS). Atherosclerosis. 2014;237(1):361-8.
21. Puri R, Nissen SE, Shao M, et al. Non-HDL cholesterol and triglycerides: Implications for coronary atheroma progression and clinical events. Arterioscler Thromb Vasc Biol. 2016;36(11):2220-8.
22. Carey VJ, Bishop L, Laranjo N, et al. Contribution of high plasma triglycerides and low high-density lipoprotein cholesterol to residual risk of coronary heart disease after establishment of low-density lipoprotein cholesterol control. Am J Cardiol. 2010;106(6):757-63.
23. Lee JS, Chang PY, Zhang Y, et al. Triglyceride and HDL-C Dyslipidemia and Risks of Coronary Heart Disease and Ischemic Stroke by Glycemic Dysregulation Status: The Strong Heart Study. Diabetes Care. 2017;40(4):529-37.
24. Jayashree S, Arindam M, Vijay KV. Genetic epidemiology of coronary artery disease: An Asian Indian perspective. J Genet. 2015;94(3):539-49.
25. Thomsen M, Varbo A, Tybjærg-Hansen A, et al. Low nonfasting triglycerides and reduced all-cause mortality: A Mendelian randomization study. Clin Chem. 2014;60(5):737-46.
26. TG and HDL Working Group of the Exome Sequencing Project, National Heart, Lung, and Blood Institute, Crosby J, Peloso GM, Auer PL, et al. Loss-of-function mutations in APOC3, triglycerides, and coronary disease. N Engl J Med. 2014;371(1):22-31.
27. Do R, Stitziel NO, Won HH, et al. Exome sequencing identifies rare LDLR and APOA5 alleles conferring risk for myocardial infarction. Nature. 2015;518(7537):102-6.
28. Iyengar SS, Puri R, Narasingan SN, et al. Lipid Association of India Expert Consensus Statement on Management of Dyslipidemia in Indians 2016: Part 1. J Assoc Physicians India. 2016;64(3):7-52.

29. Jellinger PS, Handelsman Y, Rosenblit PD, et al. American Association of Clinical Endocrinologists and American College of Endocrinology guidelines for management of dyslipidemia and prevention of cardiovascular disease. Endocr Pract. 2017;23(Suppl 2):1-87.
30. Jayaram S, Jain MM, Naikawadi AA, et al. Comparative evaluation of the efficacy, safety, and tolerability of rosuvastatin 10 mg with atorvastatin 10 mg in adult patients with hypercholesterolaemia: the first Indian study. J Indian Med Assoc. 2004;102(1):48-50, 52.
31. Deedwania PC, Gupta M, Stein M, et al.; IRIS Study Group. Comparison of rosuvastatin versus atorvastatin in South-Asian patients at risk of coronary heart disease (from the IRIS Trial). Am J Cardiol. 2007;99(11):1538-43.
32. Pu J, Romanelli R, Zhao B, Dyslipidemia in special ethnic populations. Cardiol Clin. 2015;33(2):325-33.
33. Kaul U, Varma J, Kahali D, et al. Post-marketing study of clinical experience of atorvastatin 80 mg vs 40 mg in Indian patients with acute coronary syndrome—a randomized, multi-centre study (CURE-ACS). J Assoc Physicians India. 2013;61(2):97-101.

11
CHAPTER

Lipodystrophies: Endocrine Effects

Emmy Grewal, Rajat Gupta

ABSTRACT

Lipodystrophies are a group of heterogeneous disorders characterized by selective loss of body fat and predisposition to insulin resistance and its metabolic and endocrine complications. They are subclassified depending on the degree of fat loss and whether the disorder is genetic or acquired. The extent of fat loss determines the severity of associated metabolic complications such as diabetes mellitus, hypertriglyceridemia, polycystic ovary syndrome, and hepatic steatosis. The severity of the metabolic abnormalities is usually proportional to the extent of fat loss, patients with congenital and acquired generalized lipodystrophies develop complications at early ages. Localized lipodystrophy does not have associated metabolic derangements and it is mostly a cosmetic problem. Management of lipodystrophy focuses on preventing and treating endocrine and metabolic complications. Patients with generalized lipodystrophy have markedly reduced serum leptin levels and metreleptin replacement therapy has been used successfully in such patients to improve metabolic profile.

INTRODUCTION

Adipose tissue is an important endocrine organ that regulates energy homeostasis, food intake and satiety as well as insulin signaling, glucose and lipid metabolism. It secretes several adipokines, which regulate glucose and lipid metabolism, insulin sensitivity, energy homeostasis, inflammatory activity, oxidative stress, and endothelial functions. Several enzymes expressed in the adipose tissue such as peroxisome proliferator-activated receptor-alpha (PPAR-α), PPAR-γ, 11-β hydroxysteroid dehydrogenase (11β-HSD), aromatase, and steroid sulfatase are involved in various hormonal pathways, as discussed in the chapter "Adipose tissue as an endocrine organ". Therefore, lipodystrophies are associated with a myriad of endocrine manifestations.

Lipodystrophies are heterogeneous disorders characterized by selective deficiency of adipose tissue in the absence of nutritional deprivation or catabolic state.

This can occur either in the presence or absence of metabolic abnormalities, and with diverse clinical presentations encountered in endocrine practice. While generalized forms of lipodystrophy are often diagnosed during childhood or adolescence, some forms of lipodystrophy, particularly familial partial lipodystrophy, may bear some resemblance to common metabolic disorders like obesity and syndromes of insulin resistance.[1] The loss of body fat can result from underlying genetic defects (genetic lipodystrophies including autosomal recessive or dominant subtypes) or from autoimmune mechanisms (acquired lipodystrophies including generalized or partial subtypes) or drugs [e.g., highly active antiretroviral therapy (HAART) induced partial lipodystrophy in human immunodeficiency virus (HIV) infected patients or localized lipodystrophies from insulin and other injected drugs]. The localized lipodystrophies and lipodystrophy in HIV-infected patients are the most prevalent subtype of lipodystrophies while the other genetic and acquired lipodystrophies are quite rare.[2]

Partial and generalized lipodystrophies predispose the patients to insulin resistance and its associated endocrine complications such as diabetes mellitus, hypertriglyceridemia, hepatic steatosis, polycystic ovary syndrome (PCOS), and acanthosis nigricans. The extent of fat loss determines the severity of metabolic and other complications. Major causes of mortality include heart disease (cardiomyopathy, heart failure, myocardial infarction, arrhythmia), liver disease (liver failure, gastrointestinal hemorrhage, hepatocellular carcinoma), kidney failure, acute pancreatitis (from extreme hypertriglyceridemia and chylomicronemia), and sepsis.[3,4]

Lipodystrophy syndromes are a rare body of diseases for which prevalence is currently estimated to be 1.3–4.7 cases/million. Although the molecular basis of lipodystrophy has remarkably revealed a wide heterogeneity with respect to the underlying genes and their biological pathways, a common characteristic in most lipodystrophies is that of insulin resistance. Patients with generalized lipodystrophy have extremely low serum levels of adipocytokines such as leptin and adiponectin, whereas serum leptin and adiponectin levels in those with partial lipodystrophies can range from low to high. Marked hypoleptinemia may induce excessive appetite that further exacerbates insulin resistance.[5] Leptin has also emerged as a significant factor in the regulation of bone mass. In humans, states of energy deprivation with low serum leptin have been associated with low-bone mass. Leptin affects bone metabolism through direct effects on osteocytes and chondrocytes; and indirectly by its effects on hormones such as estrogen, cortisol, insulin-like growth factor-1 (IGF-1), and parathyroid hormone. Patients with lipodystrophy have low leptin levels which decreases bone density, but they often have comorbid insulin resistance that may preserve bone density due to the high insulin and IGF-1 levels present.[6]

AN OVERVIEW OF LIPODYSTROPHY TYPES

Inherited Lipodystrophies

These forms of lipodystrophies are rare and have distinct phenotypic expressions. These include the following.

Congenital Generalized Lipodystrophy (Berardinelli–Seip Syndrome)

This autosomal recessive disorder has prevalence of about 1 in 10 million. It is recognized at birth due to complete absence of adipose tissue and hence generalized muscular appearance. In later age, patient usually develops acanthosis nigricans, fatty liver, PCOS, hypertriglyceridemia, and diabetes mellitus. Only a few patients develop diabetes during infancy, but most often diabetes appears during the teenage years or later. Later during childhood, acanthosis nigricans develops on extensive areas of the skin. Children usually have a voracious appetite and accelerated growth. Most common mutation is found at chromosome 9q34, involving gene 1-acylglycerol-3-phosphate O-acyltransferase 2 (*AGPAT2*). Aberrant AGPAT2 enzyme results in reduced synthesis of triglycerides in adipose tissues and hence causing lipodystrophy.[7]

Familial Partial Lipodystrophy (Dunnigan Syndrome)

This is a form of autosomal dominant dystrophy which manifests around puberty. This is characterized by loss of subcutaneous fat from limbs, hips, and buttocks. This form of lipodystrophy is frequently associated with metabolic complications including coronary heart disease. Most cases result from mutations in *LMNA* (lamin A/C) or PPAR-γ gene.

Lipodystrophy Associated with Mandibuloacral Dysplasia

This autosomal recessive form of lipodystrophy is characterized by mandibular and clavicular hypoplasia. Fat loss can involve only arms and legs, or it can be generalized in some cases.

Acquired Lipodystrophies

Acquired Generalized Lipodystrophy (Lawrence Syndrome)

Lawrence syndrome is an acquired disorder associated with autoimmune disorders. It shares many features with CGL including early onset of loss of body fat, insulin resistance and hypertriglyceridemia. In addition to reduction of subcutaneous fat, adipose tissue is lost from palms, soles, and intra-abdominal area.

Acquired Partial Lipodystrophy (Barraquer–Simons Syndrome)

The onset of APL in most patients occurs before the age of 15 years. Fat loss occurs gradually in a symmetric fashion, first affecting the face and then spreading downward. Most patients lose fat from the face, neck, upper extremities, and trunk, and subcutaneous fat from the lower abdomen and legs is spared. However, approximately one-fifth of the patients develop membranoproliferative glomerulonephritis, and have low levels of complement 3 and a circulating autoantibody called complement 3-nephritic factor.[8]

Insulin-induced Lipodystrophy

Insulin-induced lipodystrophy is an acquired partial lipodystrophy. Lipohypertrophy and lipoatrophy are the two main dermatological complications of subcutaneous insulin injections. Lipoatrophy is the loss of subcutaneous fat at the site of insulin injection and manifests as a visible depression. It is an immunological response to insulin aggregates, in the presence of high circulating titers of anti-insulin autoantibodies. Lipoatrophy was more prevalent in the pre-human insulin era due to the use of animal insulin. Since the introduction of recombinant human insulin and analogue insulins, lipoatrophy has become less common. On the other hand, lipohypertrophy still remains a serious local problem of insulin therapy. Lipohypertrophy is characterized by a benign tumor-like swelling of the fibrofatty tissue at the injection site secondary to lipogenic effect of insulin therapy and repetitive microtrauma. The worldwide Injection Technique Questionnaire study survey indicated that lipohypertrophy was self-reported by 29% of patients and was found by physical examination in 30.8% by healthcare providers.[9] Lipohypertrophy develops as patients inject repeatedly at the same site and occurs more frequently on both sides of the umbilicus or on midthigh, as these are commonly used sites for injection and are easily reached and convenient for patients. As injections in lipohypertrophic areas are relatively painless, patients tend to inject in the same area again and again rather than move to a new painful site. This is clinically important as insulin absorption from such sites becomes erratic leading to higher glycemic variability and unpredictable hypoglycemic episodes. Other possible risk factors for lipohypertrophy are longer duration of insulin therapy, high number of insulin injections, and reuse of needles with a significant increase if used more than five times. When large areas are involved, it can be cosmetically unsightly and socially embarrassing for patients.

Injection sites should be examined and palpated by healthcare professionals at least annually and more frequently in case of erratic glycemic control. The best current preventative and therapeutic strategies for lipohypertrophy include rotation of injection sites. Patients should be educated regarding proper injection techniques, avoiding reuse of needles, rotating injection sites and detection as well as prevention of lipohypertrophy. Individuals should be advised not to inject into areas of lipohypertrophy until abnormal tissue returns to normal, which will take several months or even years.

HAART-induced Lipodystrophy in HIV-infected Patients

Human immunodeficiency infection and treatment, both are associated with several endocrinopathies like adrenal insufficiency, hypogonadism, diabetes, thyroid dysfunction, osteopenia and osteoporosis, AIDS wasting syndrome and HIV lipodystrophy. One of the common endocrine manifestations of HIV infection is HIV-associated lipodystrophy syndrome (HALS), the most common form of partial lipodystrophy. First reported in 1998, HALS mainly develops in patients infected with HIV who are receiving highly active antiretroviral therapy (HAART), though it has been reported in HAART-naïve patients. Importantly, HALS is different from and independent of HIV-related wasting, that refers to the fat loss caused by either HIV-infection itself or by opportunistic infections and cancers. HIV-related wasting involves not only adipose tissue but also other tissues, such as muscle tissue. The pattern of fat loss is also different from HALS as it is more generalized.

The HALS patients may experience lipoatrophy, lipohypertrophy, or a combination of both.[10] HIV-associated lipodystrophy is clinically characterized by progressive and selective thinning of the subcutaneous fat tissue in the cheeks, arms, and legs; with or without accumulation of fat in dorsocervical area (buffalo hump), abdomen, suprapubic area, under the axilla, and over the anterior aspect of neck as double chin. The fat loss worsens with ongoing HAART therapy and does not reverse on discontinuation of protease inhibitors. The physical signs of lipodystrophy usually appear progressively, increasing in severity for a period of 18-24 months and then apparently stabilizing for at least 2 years. HALS increases the risk for insulin resistance, diabetes mellitus, dyslipidemia, and cardiovascular disease. Dyslipidemia is characterized by increase in triglyceride levels and low density lipoprotein (LDL) cholesterol, particularly small dense LDL. High density lipoprotein (HDL) cholesterol levels are decreased while there is an increase in lipoprotein (a), apolipoprotein B, C-III, E and H.[11]

Risk factors for HALS include older age, female sex, high baseline body fat, and greater severity of HIV infection, increased viral load, low-CD4 count, and coinfection with hepatitis C virus.[12] The development of lipodystrophy syndrome is influenced by the type of antiretroviral therapy and the duration of treatment. Nucleoside reverse transcriptase inhibitors (NRTIs), particularly zidovudine and stavudine are strongly associated with the loss of peripheral subcutaneous fat, whereas protease inhibitors (PIs) are more closely associated with localized fat accumulation, hypertriglyceridemia, and insulin resistance.[13] The NRTIs have been shown to impair adipocyte differentiation either through mitochondrial toxicity or by induction of genes that inhibit adipogenesis. On the other hand, PIs impair adipocyte differentiation through alterations in the expression of the transcription factor sterol responsive element binding protein-1c, impairment of adipokine regulation, and adipocyte apoptosis mediated by proinflammatory cytokines such as tumor necrosis factor-alpha (TNF-α) and interleukin-6 (IL-6).

DIAGNOSIS AND DIFFERENTIAL DIAGNOSIS

The diagnosis of lipodystrophy is based on history, physical examination, body composition, and metabolic status. The cardinal feature of lipodystrophy is the selective loss of subcutaneous adipose tissue. The adipose tissue abnormalities that characterize various lipodystrophy syndromes are enlisted in table 1. Lipodystrophies should be considered in the differential diagnosis of patients presenting with endocrine and metabolic disorders such as early diabetes, severe hypertriglyceridemia, hepatic steatosis, hepatosplenomegaly, acanthosis nigricans, and PCOS. The clinical features that should raise suspicion toward a diagnosis of lipodystrophy syndromes are enumerated in box 1.

A thorough physical examination of "lean" patients with these metabolic complications to look for evidence of fat loss should clinch the diagnosis. Some patients of familial partial lipodystrophy may present with excess subcutaneous fat deposition in various anatomic regions such as face and neck along with truncal obesity and may resemble patients with Cushing's syndrome. Female patients can present with delayed puberty, menstrual irregularities, infertility, hirsutism, or PCOS.

SECTION 2: Endocrine Aspects of Lipidology

TABLE 1 Classification, clinical features, and molecular basis of genetic and acquired lipodystrophies

Type	Subtype	Clinical features	Pathogenic mechanism
Autosomal recessive: Congenital generalized lipodystrophy (CGL)	• CGL 1/2/3/4	• Lack of metabolically active adipose tissue since birth • Generalized muscular appearance • Develop metabolic complications	• Various enzymes involved like AGPAT, *BSCL2*, Caveolin 1, PTRF involved in adipocytic differentiation
Autosomal dominant: Familial partial lipodystrophy (FPL)	• FPLD 1–5	• Loss of subcutaneous fat from the extremities, frequently associated with metabolic complications	• Mutations in LMNA or PPAR gamma gene
Mandibuloacral dysplasia (MAD)	• Type A (*LMNA*) • Type B (*ZMPSTE24*)	• Loss of subcutaneous fat from the extremities and trunk • Skeletal abnormalities such as mandibular and clavicular hypoplasia and acro-osteolysis	• Mutations in lamin A/C (*LMNA*) or zinc metalloproteinase (*ZMPSTE24*) which disrupts nuclear function
Lipodystrophy in HIV-infected patients	• PI-induced • NRTI-induced	• Loss of subcutaneous fat from the face and extremities and excess fat deposition in the neck and abdomen	• PI may inhibit ZMPSTE24 and/or cause dysregulation of transcription factors involved in adipogenesis • NRTI may inhibit mitochondrial polymerase- and cause mitochondrial toxicity
Acquired partial lipodystrophy	• Autoimmune • MPGN-associated • Idiopathic	• Loss of subcutaneous fat from the face, neck, upper limbs and trunk, sparing the lower abdomen, and lower limbs	• Low serum complement-3 levels, complement 3 nephritic factor, suggest autoimmune-mediated loss of adipose tissue
Acquired generalized lipodystrophy	• Autoimmune • Panniculitis-associated • Idiopathic	• Generalized loss of fat associated with tender subcutaneous nodules, autoimmune or other diseases	• Immune-mediated loss of adipose tissue
Localized lipodystrophy	• Drug-induced • Panniculitis-induced • Pressure-induced • Centrifugal Idiopathic	• Loss of subcutaneous fat from small areas of the body	• Multiple mechanisms including local drug-induced, immune-mediated, or pressure-induced atrophy of adipose tissue

AGPAT, 1-acylglycerol-3-phosphate O-acyltransferase; BSCL, Berardinelli-Seip congenital lipodystrophy; HIV, human immunodeficiency virus; LMNA, lamin A/C; MPGN, membranoproliferative glomerulonephritis; NRTI, nucleoside reverse transcriptase inhibitors; PI, protease inhibitors; PTRF, polymerase I and transcript release factor; ZMPSTE24, zinc metalloproteinase.

> **BOX 1**   **Clinical characteristics that increase the suspicion of lipodystrophy**
>
> *Clinical features that increase the suspicion of lipodystrophy*
>
> **Essential features**
> - Generalized or regional absence of body fat
>
> **Physical features**
> - Failure to thrive (infants and children)
> - Prominent muscles
> - Prominent veins (phlebomegaly)
> - Severe acanthosis nigricans
> - Eruptive xanthomata
> - Cushingoid appearance
> - Acromegaloid appearance
> - Progeroid (premature aging) appearance
>
> **Comorbid conditions**
> - Diabetes mellitus with high insulin requirements
>   - ≥200 U/day
>   - ≥2 U/kg/day
>   - Requiring U-500 insulin
> - Severe hypertriglyceridemia
>   - ≥500 mg/dL with or without therapy
>   - ≥250 mg/dL despite diet and medical therapy
>   - History of acute pancreatitis secondary to hypertriglyceridemia
> - Nonalcoholic steatohepatitis in a nonobese individual
> - Early-onset cardiomyopathy
> - Polycystic ovary syndrome
>
> **Other historical clues**
> - Autosomal dominant or recessive pattern of similar physical features or metabolic complications
> - Significant hyperphagia (may manifest as irritability/aggression in infants/children)

Presence of muscular appearance and severe insulin resistance in thin lean patients point toward diagnosis of lipodystrophy in PCOS patients. Congenital generalized lipodystrophy may present with accelerated growth, advanced bone age in childhood, acromegaloid features in adults, insulin resistance and acanthosis, hypogonadism or hyperandrogenic features.

Table 2 enlists the various hormonal and systemic features of different lipodystrophies. The other endocrine disorders which may feature in the differential diagnosis of endocrinopathies include uncontrolled diabetes, metabolic syndrome, Cushing's syndrome, acromegaly, PCOS, thyrotoxicosis, adrenal insufficiency, and multiple lipomatosis.

Diagnosis of lipodystrophy is mainly clinical, but laboratory tests can provide additional supportive evidence. All patients except those with localized lipodystrophy should be tested for glucose intolerance, serum lipids, liver function, and hyperuricemia and should be screened for cardiovascular and reproductive dysfunction. There are no defined serum leptin levels that establish or rule out the diagnosis of lipodystrophy, but leptin levels may predict response to metreleptin replacement therapy. Additional information on fat loss may be provided by skinfold thickness measurement, dual-energy X-ray absorptiometry, and a whole-body T1-weighted magnetic resonance imaging. Analysis of serum complement 3 and 4, complement 3 nephritic factor, and urinalysis for proteinuria should be conducted in patients with APL and AGL. Pubertal assessment and gonadal functions may need to be monitored in women presenting with menstrual disturbances or hyperandrogenic features. Genetic testing should be considered in at-risk family members.[8]

SECTION 2: Endocrine Aspects of Lipidology

TABLE 2 Hormonal and other manifestations of lipodystrophies

	Presentation	Subtypes
Physical appearance	Acromegaloid appearance	CGL
	Cushingoid appearance	FPL
	Progeroid appearance	Progeroid syndromes
Growth	Accelerated growth	CGL 1 and 2
	Delayed growth and short stature	CGL 3
Puberty	Precocious puberty	CGL 1 and 2
	Delayed puberty	FPL
Dermatological	Eruptive xanthomas	CGL, AGL, FPL
	Acanthosis nigricans	CGL, AGL, FPL
	Subcutaneous nodules (panniculitis)	AGL
Abdominal examination	Hepatosplenomegaly	CGL, AGL, FPL
Appetite	Hyperphagia	CGL, AGL, FPL
Insulin sensitivity	Insulin resistance	CGL, AGL, FPL
Glucose homeostasis	Diabetes, high insulin dose	CGL, AGL, FPL
Lipid parameters	High triglycerides, low HDL cholesterol	CGL, AGL, FPL
Reproductive dysfunction	Menstrual irregularities, hyperandrogenism, hirsutism, subfertility, PCOS	CGL, AGL, FPL
	Hypogonadism	Cockayne syndrome
	Hypogonadism and cryptorchidism	MDPL
Pancreatitis	Acute pancreatitis (hypertriglyceridemia)	CGL, AGL, FPL
Hepatic	NAFLD	CGL, AGL, FPL, APL
Renal	MPGN	APL
	Diabetic nephropathy	CGL, AGL, FPL, APL
Cardiac	Cardiomyopathy, HTN, CVD	CGL, AGL, FPL

AGL, acquired generalized lipodystrophy; APL, acquired partial lipodystrophy; CGL, congenital generalized lipodystrophy; CVD, cardiovascular disease; FPL, familial partial lipodystrophy; HTN, hypertension; MDPL, mandibular hypoplasia-deafness-progeroid features syndrome; MPGN, membranoproliferative glomerulonephritis; NAFLD, nonalcoholic fatty liver disease; PCOS, polycystic ovary syndrome; HDL, high density lipoprotein.

MANAGEMENT OF LIPODYSTROPHY

There is still no curative treatment for the morphological changes induced by lipodystrophy. The treatment of lipodystrophy aims to ameliorate both the endocrine and metabolic disturbances and pathological changes in fat distribution. Proper counseling of the parents as far as pathogenesis and expected course of the type of lipodystrophy is critical for allaying stress and psychological sequelae in children affected with lipodystrophies. Parents should provide support to affected children to help them adjust among their friends and classmates.

General Approach: Lifestyle Modification

Diet and Nutritional Therapy

The cornerstone of therapy for metabolic complications of lipodystrophy is diet. For lack of clinical trial evidence, all patients are advised to consume energy-restricted diet, to lower triglycerides and glucose, but dietary restriction is challenging to achieve. Patients should follow diets with balanced macronutrient composition i.e. 50–60% of total caloric intake from carbohydrates, 20–30% from fat, and approximately 20% from protein. Simple sugars should be restricted in preference for high-fiber complex carbohydrates. Dietary fat should be primarily cis-mono-unsaturated fats and long-chain ω-3 fatty acids. In extremely hypertriglyceridemic infants, medium-chain triglyceride based formula may help.[14] During acute pancreatitis, bowel rest followed by a very-low-fat (20 g) diet, should be used.

Exercise

Although few studies have examined the effect of exercise on congenital lipodystrophies, exercise has been shown to benefit patients with HALS. Increased physical activity, especially aerobic training, can lower insulin resistance. Resistance training can increase total lean mass and decrease total, truncal, and limb fat as well as reduce triglyceride levels, increase HDL cholesterol levels, and improve peripheral insulin sensitivity. Patients with familial partial lipodystrophy (FPL) with concomitant cardiomyopathy however may avoid strenuous exercise.[15] Contact sports should be avoided in patients with severe hepatosplenomegaly and CGL patients with lytic bone lesions.

Management of Endocrine and Metabolic Complications

No controlled clinical trials have been conducted to help guide drug therapy for the endocrine manifestation of lipodystrophies and the approach needs to be individualized after careful assessment.

Lipids should be managed in accordance with international guidelines for the general population, with statins as first-line therapy.[16] Statins and fibrates should be used with caution due to increased risk of myopathy, especially in the presence of known myositis or muscular dystrophy. Fibrates and/or long-chain ω-3 fatty acids should be used if triglycerides ≥500 mg/dL and maybe considered for triglycerides ≥200 mg/dL. Additional lipid-lowering drugs have not been studied in patients with lipodystrophy.

Metformin should be the first-line therapy for diabetes. However, metformin may worsen peripheral fat loss, and should be used with caution in lipoatrophic patients. In patients with partial lipodystrophy, thiazolidinediones may improve HbA1c, triglycerides, hepatic volume, and steatosis, but can potentially increase unwanted fat deposition in nonlipodystrophic regions. Whether thiazolidinediones should be the therapy of choice in FPL patients with PPARG mutations is not clear.[17] For many patients with generalized lipodystrophy, insulin therapy is needed, and insulin dose requirements may be very high. If the daily dose of insulin exceeds 200 U, concentrated insulin should be used. Insulin glargine and degludec kinetics may be altered when injected in lipodystrophic areas because their long duration of action requires subcutaneous fat.[18,19] Patients with generalized lipodystrophy may have to take insulin by intramuscular routes for the lack of subcutaneous fat. Angiotensin-converting enzyme inhibitors or angiotensin receptor blockers are first-line treatments for hypertension in patients with diabetes.

Metreleptin

Lipodystrophies are characterized by low levels of adipocyte-derived hormones like leptin; and leptin therapy remains a major therapeutic target in patients with lipodystrophies. Currently, metreleptin (recombinant human methionyl leptin) is the only drug approved specifically for generalized forms of congenital and acquired lipodystrophies. Leptin replacement therapy has been shown to be effective in improving glycemic control, lipid profile, and liver function as well as decreasing ectopic fat deposition in liver and skeletal muscle.[20,21]

Metreleptin decreases hyperphagia, frequently leading to weight loss. Reduced food intake is at least partially responsible for many of the metabolic improvements. In various studies, metreleptin markedly improved fasting glucose and triglyceride levels within 1 week[22] and lowered HbA1c by 2% after 1 year. Metreleptin also decreased LDL and total cholesterol, but did not change HDL cholesterol.[22,23] Metreleptin reduced hepatic steatosis, serum transaminases, and nonalcoholic steatohepatitis (NASH) scores within 6–12 months.[24] In females, metreleptin normalized gonadotropin secretion, leading to normal progression of puberty, normalization of menstrual periods, and improved fertility.[25] Leptin administration for 12 months decreased lean body mass and fat content, decreased energy expenditure and caloric intake, but had no impact on bone mineralization, bone resorption, or bone metabolism biomarkers in patients with lipodystrophy.[26] The response to metreleptin in partial lipodystrophy is less robust than in generalized lipodystrophy and may be considered for hypoleptinemic (leptin <4 ng/mL) patients with partial lipodystrophy and severe metabolic derangements (HbA1c >8% and/or triglycerides >500 mg/dL).[23]

CONCLUSION

Lipodystrophies are a heterogeneous group of conditions in which there is either a congenital or acquired loss of adipose tissue deposits. Lipodystrophies may present with myriad metabolic and endocrine features including insulin resistance, hypertriglyceridemia, diabetes with high insulin dose requirements, hyperandrogenism or PCOS, acromegaloid or Cushingoid features, nonalcoholic fatty liver disease or cardiovascular disease. Differentiating lipodystrophy syndromes from other more common endocrinopathies such as type 2 diabetes, metabolic syndrome or PCOS is important as it has therapeutic implications. Diabetes management in lipodystrophy syndromes can be challenging as the insulin dose requirements may be significantly high. Insulin sensitizers such as metformin and pioglitazone are often used. Although, leptin treatment can have impressive therapeutic effects, more work is needed to further explore ways to ameliorate the degree of fat loss as well as pathological fat accumulation in patients with lipodystrophy and to prevent and treat the concomitant metabolic disturbances as well as the associated long-term morbidity and mortality. In addition, prevention of insulin injection-associated lipodystrophy and its early identification are important in general clinical practice among diabetic patients using insulin.

REFERENCES

1. Handelsman Y, Oral EA, Bloomgarden ZT, et al. The clinical approach to the detection of lipodystrophy – an AACE consensus statement. Endocr Pract. 2013;19(1):107-16.
2. Garg A, Misra A. Lipodystrophies: Rare disorders causing metabolic syndrome. Endocrinol Metab Clin North Am. 2004;33(2):305-31.
3. Lupsa BC, Sachdev V, Lungu AO, et al. Cardiomyopathy in congenital and acquired generalized lipodystrophy: A clinical assessment. Medicine (Baltimore). 2010;89(4):245-50.
4. Garg A. Clinical review: Lipodystrophies: Genetic and acquired body fat disorders. J Clin Endocrinol Metab. 2011;96(11):3313-25.
5. Haque WA, Shimomura I, Matsuzawa Y, et al. Serum adiponectin and leptin levels in patients with lipodystrophies. J Clin Endocrinol Metab. 2002;87(5):2395-8.
6. Upadhyay J, Farr OM, Mantzoros CS. The role of leptin in regulating bone metabolism. Metabolism. 2015;64(1):105-13.
7. Garg A. Acquired and inherited lipodystrophies. N Engl J Med. 2004;350(12):1220-34.
8. Brown RJ, Araujo-Vilar D, Cheung PT, et al. The diagnosis and management of lipodystrophy syndromes: A multi-society practice guideline. J Clin Endocrinol Metab. 2016;101(12):4500-11.
9. Frid AH, Hirsch LJ, Menchior AR, et al. Worldwide Injection Technique Questionnaire Study: Injecting complications and the role of the professional. Mayo Clin Proc. 2016;91(9):1224-30.
10. Chen D, Misra A, Garg A. Clinical review 153: Lipodystrophy in human immunodeficiency virus-infected patients. J Clin Endocrinol Metab. 2002;87(11):4845-56.
11. Carr A, Samaras K, Burton S, et al. A syndrome of peripheral lipodystrophy, hyperlipidaemia and insulin resistance in patients receiving HIV protease inhibitors. AIDS. 1998;12(7):F51-8.
12. Kotler DP. Hepatitis C, human immunodeficiency virus and metabolic syndrome: Interactions. Liver Int. 2009;29(4):38-46.
13. Shlay JC, Sharma S, Peng G, et al. Community Programs for Clinical Research on AIDS (CPCRA); International Network for Strategic Initiatives in Global HIV Trials (INSIGHT). The effect of individual antiretroviral drugs on body composition in hiv infected persons initiating highly active antiretroviral therapy. J Acquir Immune Defic Syndr. 2009; 51(3):298-304.
14. Wilson DE, Chan IF, Stevenson KB, et al. Eucaloric substitution of medium chain triglycerides for dietary long chain fatty acids in acquired total lipodystrophy: Effects on hyperlipoproteinemia and endogenous insulin resistance. J Clin Endocrinol Metab. 1983;57(3):517-23.
15. Pasotti M, Klersy C, Pilotto A, et al. Long-term outcome and risk stratification in dilated cardio-laminopathies. J Am Coll Cardiol. 2008;52(15):1250-60.
16. Jellinger PS, Smith DA, Mehta AE, et al. American Association of Clinical Endocrinologists' guidelines for management of dyslipidemia and prevention of atherosclerosis. Endocr Pract. 2012;18(suppl 1):1-78.
17. Tan GD, Savage DB, Fielding BA, et al. Fatty acid metabolism in patients with PPAR gamma mutations. J Clin Endocrinol Metab. 2008;93(1):4462-70.
18. Karges B, Boehm BO, Karges W. Early hypoglycaemia after accidental intramuscular injection of insulin glargine. Diabet Med. 2005;22(10):1444-45.
19. Bolli GB, Owens DR. Insulin glargine. Lancet. 2000;356(9228):443-5.
20. Oral EA, Simha V, Ruiz E, et al. Leptin-replacement therapy for lipodystrophy. N Engl J Med. 2002;346(8):570-8.
21. Oral EA, Chan JL. Rationale for leptin-replacement therapy for severe lipodystrophy. Endocr Pract. 2010;16(2):324-33.

22. Ebihara K, Kusakabe T, Hirata M, et al. Efficacy and safety of leptin-replacement therapy and possible mechanisms of leptin actions in patients with generalized lipodystrophy. J Clin Endocrinol Metab. 2007; 92(2):532-41.
23. Diker-Cohen T, Cochran E, Gorden P, et al. Partial and generalized lipodystrophy: Comparison of baseline characteristics and response to metreleptin. J Clin Endocrinol Metab. 2015;100(5):1802-10.
24. Javor ED, Ghany MG, Cochran EK, et al. Leptin reverses nonalcoholic steatohepatitis in patients with severe lipodystrophy. Hepatology. 2005;41(4):753-60.
25. Musso C, Cochran E, Javor E, et al. The long-term effect of recombinant methionyl human leptin therapy on hyperandrogenism and menstrual function in female and pituitary function in male and female hypoleptinemic lipodystrophic patients. Metabolism. 2005;54(2):255-63.
26. Moran SA, Patten N, Young JR, et al. Changes in body composition in patients with severe lipodystrophy after leptin replacement therapy. Metabolism. 2004;53(4):513.

CHAPTER 12

Endovigilance in Lipid Disorders

Sunil K Kota, Sambit Das, Lalit K Meher

ABSTRACT

Various endocrine disorders are associated with significant alterations in lipid profile, with some manifesting as frank dyslipidemia. Several hormonal therapies and other drugs used to treat endocrinopathies are also associated with clinically significant changes in lipids. Dyslipidemia in endocrine disease can contribute to increased cardiovascular risk and increase morbidity and mortality. Therefore, lipid vigilance is needed in the endocrine clinic. At the same time, abnormalities in lipid parameters should prompt a clinical assessment for endocrine disorders including diabetes, metabolic syndrome, hypothyroidism, polycystic ovary syndrome (PCOS), Cushing's syndrome, acromegaly and hypogonadism, and further evaluation is needed if there are clinical indicators of endocrine abnormalities. Dyslipidemia may in fact be considered a clinical clue to endocrine disorders. Treatment of underlying endocrine disease may lead to amelioration of hyperlipidemia/dyslipidemia and improve general metabolic and cardiovascular health. At the same time, some patients with endocrinopathies may require additional lipid-lowering drugs for cardiovascular risk reduction.

INTRODUCTION

Various endocrine disorders are associated with significant alterations in lipid profile, with some even manifesting as frank dyslipidemia. Several hormonal therapies and other drugs used to treat endocrinopathies are also associated with clinically significant changes in lipids.[1] The effects on lipid metabolism can manifest in the form of alteration in plasma lipid and lipoprotein levels. Some of these are protective, while others are detrimental for the development of atherosclerotic cardiovascular disease.[1] Additionally, some hypolipidemic drugs have impact on endocrine function as well. Dyslipidemia secondary to endocrinopathies is often amenable to treatment by addressing the core hormonal imbalance, while some patients may need hypolipidemic/lipid-lowering drugs therapy. In the current chapter, we shall outline the significance, causes, and evaluation of lipid abnormalities secondary to endocrinopathies and the therapies used. We highlight upon the need to keep an endocrine vigilance in patients presenting with dyslipidemia as some of these may be related to underlying disorders of the endocrine system, with significant implications in management.

DEFINITION AND TYPES OF DYSLIPIDEMIA

Dyslipidemias are characterized by an abnormal amount of lipids and lipoproteins [e.g., total cholesterol, low-density lipoprotein cholesterol, high-density lipoprotein cholesterol, very low density lipoprotein cholesterol, apolipoprotein B, and lipoprotein(a)] in the blood. The most common dyslipidemia seen in general practice is hyperlipidemia or abnormal elevation of lipids including cholesterol (hypercholesterolemia) or triglycerides (hypertriglyceridemia) or both (combined dyslipidemia). Dyslipidemia has been long considered to be a significant contributor to the pathogenesis of atherosclerosis and atherosclerotic cardiovascular disease. Since, it is a modifiable cardiovascular risk factor that is amenable to treatment, its identification and management can have significant impact on both morbidity and mortality, as has been documented in seminal long-term trials of statins and other lipid-lowering drugs. In addition, some forms of dyslipidemia, especially significant elevations in triglycerides, may predispose to acute pancreatitis.

Hyperlipidemia may be familial (primary) resulting from specific genetic abnormalities in lipid and/or lipoprotein metabolism or acquired (secondary) when it is caused by another underlying disorder including metabolic and endocrine diseases, lifestyle-related and dietary factors, obesity, alcohol intake, or certain drugs that affect lipid metabolism.[2] However, quite often, hyperlipidemia is idiopathic without a known underlying cause.

Hyperlipidemias can also be classified according to the type of lipids that are predominantly elevated and include hypercholesterolemia, hypertriglyceridemia, and combined hyperlipidemia. The Fredrickson's classification of hyperlipidemia, as depicted in table 1, is based on the pattern of lipids and lipoproteins on electrophoresis or ultracentrifugation.[3] This was initially described for familial hyperlipidemias, and later adopted by the World Health Organization (WHO).

EPIDEMIOLOGICAL ASSOCIATIONS

Dyslipidemia is a major risk factor for coronary heart disease (CHD). According to a WHO estimate, dyslipidemia is associated with more than half of ischemic heart disease globally and more than 4 million deaths per year.[4] The total cost associated with cardiovascular disease and stroke related to dyslipidemia includes both medical services (direct costs) as well as lost wages (indirect costs). The cost burden of cardiovascular disease and stroke is substantial, though it may vary widely around the world.[5]

As per the Indian Council of Medical Research-India Diabetes (ICMR-INDIAB) study which included sample populations from three states (Tamil Nadu, Maharashtra, and Jharkhand) and one Union Territory (Chandigarh), 79% of the adult population had abnormalities in at least one of the lipid parameters. The most

TABLE 1 Fredrickson's classification of hyperlipidemia

Hyperlipo-proteinemia	Synonyms	Defect	Increased lipoprotein fraction	Elevated lipids
Type I	a. Familial Hyperchylomicronemia	Decreased lipoprotein lipase (LPL)	Chylomicrons	Triglycerides
	b. Familial apolipoprotein CII deficiency	Altered apolipoprotein CII		
	c.	LPL inhibitor in blood		
Type II	a. Familial hypercholesterolemia	LDL receptor deficiency	LDL	Cholesterol
	b. Familial combined hyperlipidemia	Decreased LDL receptor and increased apolipoprotein B	LDL and VLDL	Triglycerides and cholesterol
Type III	Familial dysbetalipoproteinemia	Defect in apolipoprotein E2 synthesis	IDL	Triglycerides and cholesterol
Type IV	Familial hypertriglyceridemia	Increased VLDL production and decreased elimination	VLDL	Triglycerides
Type V	–	Increased VLDL production and decreased LPL	VLDL and chylomicrons	Triglycerides and cholesterol

IDL, intermediate-density lipoprotein; LDL, low-density lipoprotein; VLDL, very low-density lipoprotein.

common dyslipidemia was reduced high-density lipoprotein cholesterol (HDL-C) found in 72.3%, followed by hypertriglyceridemia in 29.5%, hypercholesterolemia in 13.9%, and elevated low-density lipoprotein cholesterol (LDL-C) levels in 11.8% cases. In general, urban residents had higher prevalence of dyslipidemia. Regional disparity exists with the highest rates of low HDL-C in Jharkhand (76.8%), hypertriglyceridemia in Chandigarh (38.6%), hypercholesterolemia (18.3%), and high LDL-C (15.8%) in Tamil Nadu. The most common risk factors for dyslipidemia included obesity, diabetes, and dysglycemia.[6]

In another cross-sectional study including urban Asian Indians, the most prevalent dyslipidemias were borderline high LDL-C greater than or equal to 100 mg/dL in 49.5% and 49.7% of men and women, low HDL-C found in 33.6% and 52.8% of men and women respectively, and high triglycerides (42.1% and 32.9% of men and women). Subjects with higher socioeconomic status, greater adiposity, and high fat intake are more prone for dyslipidemia.[7]

Only about one-third of patients on treatment are achieving their National Cholesterol Education Program (NCEP) goals. Only two-thirds of patients whose test results indicated high blood cholesterol or who were taking a cholesterol-lowering medication are being informed about their high cholesterol. Fewer than half of those persons who qualify for any kind of treatment for dyslipidemia are receiving it and even worse, less than half of patients with established cardiovascular disease are optimally

SECTION 2: Endocrine Aspects of Lipidology

treated.[8] Therefore, there is huge burden of dyslipidemia that goes undetected and untreated, thus contributing to cardiovascular morbidity and mortality due to a potentially modifiable risk factor. This calls for greater vigilance for lipid abnormalities in general clinical practice.

SECONDARY DYSLIPIDEMIA: ENDOCRINE CAUSES

As described earlier, the causes of dyslipidemia can be familial due to genetic causes,[3] secondary to other chronic disorders or drugs or idiopathic.[9] In table 2, we enlist the typical lipid abnormalities that manifest due to secondary causes. A study by Vodnala et al. concluded that nearly one-third of patients referred to a speciality clinic had an identifiable secondary condition contributing to their dyslipidemia.[9] The most common causes included excessive alcohol consumption, uncontrolled diabetes mellitus, and overt albuminuria.

Amongst endocrine causes of dyslipidemia, obesity and type 2 diabetes are the most common. In addition, dyslipidemia may be caused by overt or subclinical thyroid dysfunction, PCOS, hypogonadism, hyperprolactinemia, Cushing's syndrome, acromegaly, and growth hormone deficiency.[10] The impact of these hormonal disorders on various lipid parameters is mentioned in table 3. Lipid levels can influence the clinical course of some endocrine diseases like the occurrence of microvascular and macrovascular complications in diabetes and lipotoxicity-induced β-cell failure.[1] Similarly, puberty and menopausal status can impact lipid profiles.[10] In addition, several hormonal therapies like thyroxine replacement, glucocorticoid, growth hormone, testosterone, estrogen, androgen replacement therapies, anabolic

TABLE 2 Secondary causes of various types of dyslipidemia

Predominant lipid abnormalities	Secondary causes	
	Diseases	Drugs
High triglycerides	• Diabetes mellitus • Metabolic syndrome • Hypothyroidism • Chronic kidney disease • Nephrotic syndrome • Alcoholism • Human immunodeficiency virus infection • Autoimmune disorders • Pregnancy • Polycystic ovary disease	• Beta-blockers (especially non-beta-1 selective) • Thiazide diuretics • Glucocorticoids • Rosiglitazone • Bile acid sequestrants • Oral estrogens • Tamoxifen and raloxifene • Retinoids • Immunosuppressive drugs (cyclosporine and sirolimus) • Cyclophosphamide • Interferons • Atypical antipsychotic drugs (fluperlapine, clozapine, and olanzapine) • Protease inhibitors • L-asparaginase

Continued

Continued

Predominant lipid abnormalities	Secondary causes	
	Diseases	Drugs
High LDL-cholesterol	• Diabetes • Hypothyroidism • Chronic kidney disease • Nephrotic syndrome • Obstructive liver disease • Obstructive airway disease • Human immunodeficiency virus infection • Autoimmune disorders • Pregnancy • Polycystic ovary disease	• Amiodarone • Thiazide diuretics • Glucocorticoids • Thiazolidinediones • Fibrates (in severe hypertriglyceridemia) • Long chain ω-3 fatty acids (in severe hypertriglyceridemia) • Anabolic steroids • Some progestins • Danazol • Isotretinoin • Immunosuppressive drugs (cyclosporine) • Anabolic steroids • Progestin
Low HDL cholesterol	• Obesity • Diabetes • Hypertriglyceridemia • Cigarette smoking • Puberty (males) • Menopause • Low fat intake • Infection • Inflammation • Malignancy • Paraproteinemias	• Anabolic steroid • Danazol • Thiazolidinediones • Some statin • Fibrate • Beta-blockers (without intrinsic sympathomimetic action) • Progestin • Antipsychotics

HDL, high-density lipoprotein; LDL, low-density lipoprotein.

steroids, and oral contraceptive pills have an impact on lipid parameters.[10] The impact of various hormonal therapies on lipid profiles is depicted in table 4. Some other drugs used to treat endocrine disorders also affect the lipid profile, including ketoconazole, insulin, metformin, glitazones, incretin-based therapies, octreotide, bromocriptine, and cabergoline.[1] The endocrine aspects of dyslipidemia are discussed in detail in subsequent sections.

APPROACH TO LIPID DISORDERS FROM AN ENDOCRINE PERSPECTIVE

Primary lipid disorders are suspected when patients have the following features:
- Physical signs of dyslipidemia such as xanthelasmas, planar, tuberous or eruptive xanthomas, arcus cornealis, or lipemia retinalis
- Occurrence of dyslipidemia at young age

SECTION 2: Endocrine Aspects of Lipidology

TABLE 3 Typical lipid abnormalities in various endocrine disorders

	Total Cholesterol	LDL-C	HDL-C	Triglycerides	Lp(a)	Apo B	Apo A-I
Diabetes	N to ↑	N to ↑	↓	↑	↑	-	-
Hypothyroidism	↑	↑	N to ↑	N to ↑	↑	↑	↑
Hyperthyroidism	↓	↓	↓	Variable	↓	↓	↓
Cushing's syndrome	↑	↑	Variable	↑	N to ↑	↑	Variable
Growth hormone deficiency	Variable	Variable	↓	↑	↑	-	-
Acromegaly	↑	↑	↓	↑	N	-	-
Hyperprolactinemia	↑	↑	N to ↓	N to ↑	-	-	-
Polycystic ovary syndrome	N to ↑	↑	↓	↑	↑	-	-
Hypogonadism	↑	↑	↓	↑	↑	-	-

Apo A-I, apolipoprotein A-I; Apo B, apolipoprotein B; HDL-C, high-density lipoprotein cholesterol; LDL-C, low-density lipoprotein cholesterol; Lp(a), lipoprotein(a).

- Occurrence of premature atherosclerotic cardiovascular disease
- A family history of atherosclerotic cardiovascular disease
- Significantly elevated lipid levels, such as serum cholesterol more than 240 mg/dL or serum triglycerides more than 1,000 mg/dL.

Since endocrine diseases can cause dyslipidemia, the treating clinicians need to be vigilant of the possibility of an endocrinopathy upon encountering an abnormal lipidogram. Tests for any secondary causes of dyslipidemia including endocrinopathy should be done in most patients with newly diagnosed dyslipidemia and when a component of the lipid profile has inexplicably changed for the worse in presence of a background endocrinopathy or there are telltale symptoms and signs suggestive of any endocrine disorders.[11] One should also be suspicious of a secondary cause if a patient has a sudden development of lipid/lipoprotein abnormality or the lipid/lipoprotein profile suddenly worsens in a previously stable patient.

A thorough clinical presentation, history, and clinical examination are essential to zero in on endocrine cause of dyslipidemia. Table 5 depicts clinical presentation and signs suggestive of various endocrine disorders. Additionally, enquiry should be made regarding intake of drugs that may affect lipid health (Table 4). Different endocrine disorders have distinct lipophenotypes, as outlined earlier in table 3 and the presence of these should prompt clinical evaluation for endocrine disorders.[11] Increased LDL-C levels should raise suspicion of hypothyroidism, growth hormone deficiency, Cushing's syndrome, and intake of drugs like glucocorticoids, danazol, some progestins, anabolic steroids, growth hormone, and thiazolidinediones. Elevated triglyceride levels should raise suspicion of obesity, diabetes, hypothyroidism, Cushing's syndrome, growth hormone deficiency, lipodystrophy, and drugs like estrogen, tamoxifen, or glucocorticoids. Low HDL-C can manifest in obesity and diabetes and use of drugs like anabolic steroids, danazol, progestin, or thiazolidinediones.

TABLE 4 The lipid abnormalities following various hormonal therapies

	Growth hormone	Glucocorticoid	Levothyroxine	Testosterone	Androgen deprivation therapy	Oral estrogen	Progestins	Female HRT	Anabolic steroids
Total cholesterol	→	←	-	-	←	-	-	→	-
LDL-C	→	N to ↑	→	→	←	→	Little or No	→	←
HDL-C	N to ↑	←	←	→ or no change	←	←	→	←	→
Triglycerides	No change	N to ↑	Variable	Variable	←	→	→	←	-
Lp(a)	←	-	→	→	←	→	-	→	-

HDL-C, high-density lipoprotein cholesterol; HRT, hormone replacement therapy; LDL-C, low-density lipoprotein cholesterol; Lp(a), lipoprotein(a).

SECTION 2: Endocrine Aspects of Lipidology

TABLE 5 Clinical symptoms, signs, and investigations pertinent to various endocrinopathies in patients with dyslipidemia

Disorder	Clinical presentation	Signs	Investigations
Diabetes	Increased thirst and appetite, frequent urination, unexplained weight loss, fatigue, irritability, blurred vision, delayed wound healing, frequent infections such as gums or skin infections and vaginal infections, family history of diabetes, personal history of polycystic ovary syndrome, prediabetes or gestational diabetes	• Obesity, central obesity • Signs of insulin resistance: acanthosis nigricans and skin tags	• Glucose tolerance test • Fasting and postmeal plasma glucose • HbA1C
Hypothyroidism	Fatigue, increased sensitivity to cold, constipation, dry skin, thinning of hair, weight gain, puffy face, hoarseness, muscle weakness, muscle aches and stiffness, stiffness or swelling in joints, menorrhagia or oligomenorrhea, depression, impaired memory or forgetfulness	• Obesity, myxedema, pallor, dry skin, macroglossia, coarse facial features and dull expression, brittle dry hair with thinning of hair • Bradycardia, diastolic hypertension, pericardial effusion • Slowed speech and movements, hyporeflexia with delayed relaxation of ankle reflex, ataxia • Goiter	• T3, T4, TSH • Antithyroid peroxidase antibodies
Hyperthyroidism	Weight loss, palpitations, increased appetite, nervousness, heat intolerance, anxiety and irritability, fatigue, fine tremors, excess sweating, changes in menstrual patterns, frequent bowel movements, goiter, muscle weakness	• Tachycardia or atrial arrhythmia, systolic hypertension with wide pulse pressure • Warm, moist, smooth skin • Lid lag and stare, ophthalmopathy and dermopathy • Hand tremors, muscle weakness • Goiter—diffuse or nodules	• T3, T4, TSH • Technetium scan of thyroid

Continued

Continued

Disorder	Clinical presentation	Signs	Investigations
Hyperprolactinemia	• In females: Oligomenorrhea or amenorrhea, galactorrhea, painful intercourse due to vaginal dryness, acne and hirsutism • In males: Erectile dysfunction, decreased body and facial hair, uncommonly gynecomastia • In both sexes: Low-bone density, hypopituitarism due to sellar mass, loss of interest in sexual activity, headaches, visual disturbances, infertility	• Galactorrhea in women • Gynecomastia, alopecia and loss of muscle mass in men • Visual field defects in cases of prolactinoma, sometimes obesity in prolactinoma	• Serum prolactin • MRI sella and hypothalamus • Evaluation for other anterior pituitary hormones, if clinically indicated
Acromegaly	Enlarged hands and feet, coarsened, enlarged facial features, coarse and thickened skin, excessive sweating and body odor, skin tags, fatigue and muscle weakness, deepened, husky voice, snoring, Impaired vision, headaches, enlarged tongue, pain and limited joint mobility, menstrual cycle irregularities in women, erectile dysfunction in men	• Doughy feeling skin over the face and extremities (one of the earliest signs in acromegaly is swelling of soles and palms), thick and hard nails, deepening of creases on the forehead and nasolabial folds • Macroglossia, thick and edematous eyelids, enlargement of the lower lip and nose, wide spacing of the teeth and prognathism • Skin tags, hypertrichosis, oily skin, acanthosis nigricans, excessive sweating, galactorrhea, hypertension	• Growth hormone suppression test • IGF-1 • MRI sella
Growth hormone deficiency	Adults: Anxiety and/or depression, baldness (in men), decrease in sexual function and interest, decreased muscle mass and strength, very low energy levels, centripetal obesity, difficulty in concentrating, lower tolerance to exercise, osteoporosis	• Most patients with GH deficiency have a normal physical examination. Some patients may have reduced skeletal muscle and lean body mass but increased fat mass, mainly in the abdominal region	• Growth hormone stimulation test • MRI sella
Polycystic ovary syndrome	Infrequent, irregular or prolonged menstrual cycles, hirsutism, and occasionally severe acne and male-pattern baldness	Hirsutism, other virilizing signs, such as male pattern balding or alopecia, increased muscle mass, deepening voice, or clitoromegaly, obesity	• Testosterone, DHEAS • USG abdomen and pelvis

Continued

Continued

Disorder	Clinical presentation	Signs	Investigations
Hypogonadism in men	Erectile dysfunction, infertility, decrease in beard and body hair growth, decrease in muscle mass, development of breast tissue (gynecomastia), loss of bone mass (osteoporosis)	Gynecomastia, loss of fat mass, osteoporosis	Testosterone, LH, FSH
Cushing's syndrome	Weight gain with truncal obesity and thinning of limbs, moon face and buffalo hump, pink or purple striae on the skin of the abdomen, thighs, breasts and arms, thin and fragile skin that bruises easily, slow healing of cuts, insect bites and infections, acne. Proximal muscle weakness, depression, anxiety and irritability, loss of emotional control, cognitive difficulties, hypertension and diabetes, bone loss Women: Hirsutism, irregular or absent menses Men: Decreased libido, decreased fertility, erectile dysfunction	• Central obesity, moon facies, prominent dorsocervical and supraclavicular fat pads • Violaceous striae most commonly over the abdomen, buttocks, lower back, upper thighs, upper arms, and breasts • Ecchymosis, telangiectasia and purpura, cutaneous atrophy, increased lanugo facial hair, steroid acne (papular or pustular lesions over the face, chest, and back), acanthosis nigricans, hypertension, proximal myopathy, avascular necrosis • If glucocorticoid excess is accompanied by androgen excess, as occurs in adrenocortical carcinomas, hirsutism and male pattern balding may be present in women • Tumor compression: Galactorrhea, hypothyroidism, hypogonadism, visual field defects	• 8 AM serum cortisol. Midnight (11 PM) serum cortisol • Overnight dexamethasone suppression test • Serum ACTH • 24-hour urinary free cortisol • Low dose and high dose dexamethasone suppression tests as required • MRI sella • CECT abdomen

ACTH, adrenocorticotropic hormone; CECT, contrast-enhanced computed tomography; DHEAS, dehydroepiandrosterone sulfate; FSH, follicle-stimulating hormone; GH, growth hormone; HbA1c, hemoglobin A1C; IGF-1, insulin-like growth factor 1; LH, luteinizing hormone; MRI, magnetic resonance imaging; TSH, thyroid-stimulating hormone; USG, ultrasonography.

There are several diagnostic tests for various endocrine disorders. Some of these include routine serum tests such as fasting and postprandial plasma glucose, glycosylated hemoglobin, thyroid profile, and serum testosterone. Quite often, endocrine evaluation involves hormone suppression tests when expecting disorders of hormone excess or hormone stimulation tests when suspecting hormone deficiency states and the respective testing should be prompted by clinical indicators. For example, individuals with clinical suspicion of hypercortisolism (Cushing's syndrome) should be evaluated with overnight dexamethasone suppression test, while patients with clinical suspicion of growth hormone deficiency need growth hormone stimulation testing.[12]

Routine tests of utility in endocrine evaluation of dyslipidemias include glucose tolerance test and glycosylated hemoglobin for diabetes, thyroid function test for thyroid disorders, serum prolactin for hyperprolactinemia, serum testosterone for hypogonadism, and PCOS and serum follicle-stimulating hormone (FSH) for menopausal status. Similarly, overnight dexamethasone suppression test for Cushing's syndrome, growth hormone suppression test for acromegaly, and growth hormone stimulation tests for growth hormone deficiency (following clonidine, insulin, levodopa, etc.) are indicated if there is clinical suspicion. For further confirmation or localization purposes, specific radiologic and nuclear scintigraphy-based evaluation may be needed.[13] These include ultrasound and technetium scintigraphy for thyroid disorders, magnetic resonance imaging (MRI) brain for hyperprolactinemia, acromegaly, Cushing's syndrome, growth hormone deficiency, ultrasound abdomen for PCOS, and computed tomography (CT) abdomen for adrenal etiology of Cushing's syndrome.

ENDOCRINE VIGILANCE IN THOSE ON LONG-TERM LIPID-LOWERING DRUGS

The JUPITER trial reported a 25% increased risk of diabetes with rosuvastatin 20 mg, compared to those on placebo.[14] Since then, several meta-analyses and longitudinal population-based studies suggest that there is a 9–12% increase in risk of dysglycemia with statins.[15] The risk factors for diabetes in statin-treated persons include underlying risk for diabetes at baseline, intensity of statin therapy, adherence to lifestyle modifications, and certain genetic traits. There is a modest impact of statins on worsening hyperglycemia and hemoglobin A1C (HbA1C) levels in subjects with glucose intolerance and pre-existing diabetes. Impaired insulin sensitivity and compromised β-cell function via enhanced intracellular cholesterol uptake due to inhibition of intracellular cholesterol synthesis by statins and proinflammatory effects of statins under dysmetabolic states are some reasons.[15]

Niacin leads to a rise in glucose levels in diabetic patients. Post-hoc analysis of the Coronary Drug Project suggested increase in glucose levels even in nondiabetic subjects, leading to an increase in the risk of developing diabetes.[16] As per a meta-analysis of 11 trials with 26,340 nondiabetic participants, niacin therapy was associated with a relative risk (RR) of 1.34 [95% confidence interval (CI) 1.21–1.49] for new-onset diabetes. This translates to one additional case of diabetes per 43 (95% CI 30–70) nondiabetic individuals who are treated with niacin for 5 years. Results were consistent regardless of background statin therapy or combined therapy with laropiprant.[17,18]

Vitamin D deficiency modifies the risk of musculoskeletal symptoms after statin use. Statin-induced myalgia has been reported in 27% of subjects. Vitamin D supplementation may improve tolerance to statins.[19] However, some of the benefits of vitamin D have been attributed to placebo effect.[20]

On the other hand, colesevelam, a bile acid sequestrant, has positive effect on glycemic status with mild reduction in HbA1C.[21] This is possibly mediated through farnesoid X receptor, liver X receptor, fibroblast growth factor 19 (FGF19), and TGR5-mediated effects on intestinal glucose absorption and/or hepatic glucose metabolism. There is additional influence on incretin effects, peripheral insulin sensitivity, and energy homeostasis.[21] In addition, fenofibrate and statins have some role in improvement in diabetic microvascular complications. Fenofibrate use was associated with reduction in progression of diabetic retinopathy while statins have been found beneficial in diabetic neuropathy and nephropathy.[22]

LIPID-LOWERING EFFECTS OF ENDOCRINE DRUGS

Thyroid hormones exert their effects via thyroid hormone receptors (TRs). TRβ subtype is present on liver and it regulates cholesterol and lipoprotein metabolism. Thyroid hormone analogs (thyromimetics) activate TRβ and these are selectively taken up by liver for subsequent activation. These compounds stimulate cholesterol elimination as bile acids and cholesterol, act on hepatic LDL receptors to increase clearance of LDL-C from circulation and promote reverse cholesterol transport. They have shown retardation in atherosclerosis progression in animals. In human studies, eprotirome exerted beneficial lipid-modulating effects while devoid of thyroid hormone-related side effects with maintenance of normal hypothalamic-pituitary-thyroid feedback. In addition to statins, it reduces LDL and non-HDL-C, apolipoprotein B, and triglycerides as well as lipoprotein(a).[23] In fact, levothyroxine therapy has been associated with reduction of LDL-C and lipoprotein(a) and increase in HDL-C.[10] Some studies have revealed reduction in carotid intima media thickness following levothyroxine therapy in patients with subclinical hypothyroidism.[24]

Octreotide therapy in patients with acromegaly is associated with reduction of triglycerides, total cholesterol, LDL-C, and lipoprotein(a). However, there was no change in the small and/or dense LDL particles.[25,26] Use of dopamine agonists, such as bromocriptine or cabergoline in patients with hyperprolactinemia leads to decrease in plasma total and LDL-C levels and in some instances triglycerides as well. Cabergoline is superior to bromocriptine in terms of its effect on insulin sensitivity, atherogenic dyslipidemia, and circulating levels of other cardiovascular risk factors in hyperprolactinemia patients.[27] Growth hormone replacement leads to a decrease in total, non-HDL, and LDL-C levels without any alteration in HDL-C and triglyceride levels. Some studies have reported increase in HDL and lipoprotein(a) levels.[28]

Ketoconazole, an antifungal imidazole derivative, is used in the medical management of Cushing's syndrome. It is an inhibitor of cholesterol biosynthesis and reduces activity of 3-hydroxy-3-methylglutaryl-coenzyme A reductase. It reduces total cholesterol, intermediate-density lipoprotein cholesterol, LDL-C and apolipoprotein B levels by approximately 25%.[29] In addition, ketoconazole inhibits several cytochrome P450 enzymes and interferes with the metabolism of simvastatin, lovastatin, and atorvastatin leading to increase in their plasma concentrations and risk of myotoxicity. Pravastatin, pitavastatin, and rosuvastatin are preferred as their plasma concentrations are not significantly increased by CYP3A4 inhibitors.[29]

Thiazolidinediones have variable effect on serum lipids and lipoproteins. Both pioglitazone and rosiglitazone increase HDL levels. Rosiglitazone increases LDL-C, whereas LDL-C levels remain unchanged with pioglitazone. Although pioglitazone has been associated with a decrease in triglyceride levels, there has been a variable impact of rosiglitazone on triglycerides, ranging from a 19% decrease to 2% increase.[30] While treatment with dipeptidyl peptidase 4 inhibitors leads to a significant reduction in total cholesterol, treatment with glucagon-like peptide-1 (GLP-1) receptor agonists (RAs) were associated with modest reductions in total cholesterol, LDL-C, and triglycerides but no significant improvement in HDL-C.[31,32] Sodium-glucose linked transporter type 2 (SGLT2) inhibitors are associated with reduction in triglyceride, increase in HDL-C, and increase in LDL-C, with no change in HDL-C/LDL-C.[33] Glucagon reduces serum triglyceride levels. Metformin administration leads to reduction in serum total cholesterol, LDL-C, and triglycerides.[34] Insulin injection in diabetic subjects leads to reduction in triglycerides, where as some studies have suggested increase in HDL-C.[34]

CONCLUSION

A variety of endocrine disorders and hormonal therapies can alter lipid metabolism resulting in changes in plasma lipid and lipoprotein levels. However, often the correlation between the hormonal alterations and lipid changes is not a very clear one. The dyslipidemia associated with majority of these endocrinopathies is associated with increased risk of atherosclerotic cardiovascular disease. In presence of sudden development or worsening of dyslipidemia and clinical indicators of hormonal disorders, the clinician should be vigilant to the possibility of secondary causes of dyslipidemia. Certain historical findings, clinical features, and signs may point to coexistence of endocrine disorders or intake of related drug. This shall require appropriate investigations followed by requisite treatment for the dyslipidemia to ameliorate.

REFERENCES

1. Kalra S, Priya G. Lipocrinology—the relationship between lipids and endocrine function. Drugs Context. 2018;7:212514.
2. Chait A, Brunzell JD. Acquired hyperlipidemia (secondary dyslipoproteinemias). Endocrinol Metab Clin North Am. 1990;19(2):259-78.
3. Fredrickson Ds, Lees RS. A system for phenotyping hyperlipoproteinemia. Circulation. 1965;31:321-7.
4. World Health Organization. The World Health Report 2002—Reducing Risks, Promoting Healthy Life, 2002.
5. Palmer AJ, Valentine WJ, Roze S, et al. Overview of costs of stroke from published, incidence-based studies spanning 16 industrialized countries. Curr Med Res Opin. 2005;21:19-26.
6. Joshi SR, Anjana RM, Deepa M, et al. Prevalence of dyslipidemia in urban and rural India: the ICMR-INDIAB study. PLoS One. 2014;9:e96808.
7. Guptha S, Gupta R, Deedwania P, et al. Cholesterol lipoproteins and prevalence of dyslipidemias in urban Asian Indians: a cross sectional study. Indian Heart J. 2014;66:280-8.
8. Peterson AM, McGhan WF. Pharmacoeconomic impact of non-compliance with statins. Pharmacoeconomics. 2005;23:13-25.

SECTION 2: Endocrine Aspects of Lipidology

9. Vodnala D, Rubenfire M, Brook RD. Secondary causes of dyslipidemia. Am J Cardiol. 2012;110:823-5.
10. Feingold K, Brinton EA, Grunfeld C, et al. The Effect of Endocrine Disorders on Lipids and Lipoproteins. Endotext South Dartmouth (MA). 2015.
11. Feingold KR, Grunfeld C. Approach to the Patient with Dyslipidemia. Endotext South Dartmouth (MA). 2018.
12. Jialal I. Diagnostic Tests in Endocrinology and Diabetes: Dyslipidemias and Their Investigation. London, England: Chapman and Hall; 1994. pp. 215-27.
13. Pozzili P, Lenzi A, Clarke BL, et al. Imaging in Endocrinology. New Jersey, United States: John Wiley & Sons; 2014.
14. Ridker PM, Danielson E, Fonseca FA, et al. Rosuvastatin to prevent vascular events in men and women with elevated C-reactive protein. N Engl J Med. 2008;359:2195-207.
15. Ganda OP. Statin-induced diabetes: incidence, mechanisms, and implications. F1000 Res. 2016;5:F1000 Faculty Rev-1499.
16. Sazonov V, Maccubbin D, Sisk CM, et al. Effects of niacin on the incidence of new onset diabetes and cardiovascular events in patients with normoglycaemia and impaired fasting glucose. Int J Clin Pract. 2013;67:297-302.
17. Goldie C, Taylor AJ, Nguyen P, et al. Niacin therapy and the risk of new-onset diabetes: a meta-analysis of randomised controlled trials. Heart. 2016;102:198-203.
18. Moses AM, Howanitz J, van Gemert M, et al. Clofibrate-induced antidiuresis. J Clin Invest. 1973;52:535-42.
19. Vandenberg BF, Robinson J. Management of the patient with statin intolerance. Curr Atheroscler Rep. 2010;12:48-57.
20. Khayznikov M, Kumar A, Ping Wang P, et al. Statin Intolerance and Vitamin D Supplementation. N Am J Med Sci. 2015;7:339-40.
21. Fonseca VA, Handelsman Y, Staels B. Colesevelam lowers glucose and lipid levels in type 2 diabetes: the clinical evidence. Diabetes Obes Metab. 2010;12:384-92.
22. Leiter LA. The prevention of diabetic microvascular complications of diabetes: is there a role for lipidlowering? Diabetes Res Clin Pract. 2005;68 Suppl 2:S3-14.
23. Angelin B, Rudling M. Lipid lowering with thyroid hormone and thyromimetics. Curr Opin Lipidol. 2010;21:499-506.
24. Monzani F, Caraccio N, Kozàkowà M, et al. Effect of Thyroxin Treatment on Carotid Intima–Media Thickness (CIMT) Reduction in Patients with Subclinical Hypothyroidism (SCH): a Meta-Analysis of Clinical Trials. J Atheroscler Thromb. 2017;24:643-59.
25. Cohen R, Chanson P, Bruckert E, et al. Effects of octreotide on lipid metabolism in acromegaly. Horm Metab Res. 1992;24:397-400.
26. Arosio M, Sartore G, Rossi CM, et al. LDL physical properties, lipoprotein and Lp(a) levels in acromegalic patients. Effects of octreotide therapy. Italian Multicenter Octreotide Study Group. Atherosclerosis. 2000;151:551-7.
27. Krysiak R, Okopien B. Different effects of cabergoline and bromocriptine on metabolic and cardiovascular risk factors in patients with elevated prolactin levels. Basic Clin Pharmacol Toxicol. 2015;116:251-6.
28. Kubo T, Furujo M, Takahashi K, et al. Effects of Growth Hormone Treatment on Lipid Profiles. Indian J Pediatr. 2018;85:261-5.
29. Greenman Y. Management of Dyslipidemia in Cushing's Syndrome. Neuroendocrinology. 2010; 92(suppl 1):91-5.
30. Madan P. Effect of thiazolidinediones on lipid profile. CMAJ. 2005;173:344.
31. Monami M, Lamanna C, Desideri CM, et al. DPP-4 inhibitors and lipids: systematic review and meta-analysis. Adv Ther. 2012;29:14-25.
32. Sun F, Wu S, Wang J, et al. Effect of glucagon-like peptide-1 receptor agonists on lipid profiles among type 2 diabetes: a systematic review and network meta-analysis. Clin Ther. 2015;37:225-41.
33. Inzucchi SE, Zinman B, Wanner C, et al. SGLT-2 inhibitors and cardiovascular risk: Proposed pathways and review of ongoing outcome trials. Diab Vasc Dis Res. 2015;12:90-100.
34. Chaudhuri A, Dandona P. Effects of insulin and other antihyperglycaemic agents on lipid profiles of patients with diabetes. Diabetes Obes Metab. 2011;13:869-79.

SECTION 3

Management Issues in Lipocrinology

CHAPTER 13

Lipid-lowering Drugs in the Management of Endocrinopathy

Om J Lakhani, Subhodik Pramanik

ABSTRACT

Lipid-lowering drugs have been traditionally used for improving lipid parameters and cardiovascular risk. But due to pleotropic effect of these agents, many of them have role in the management of endocrinopathies, either in the form of normalizing hormone levels or preventing complications. Cholestyramine, a bile acid sequestrant, binds thyroxine in the intestine and is therefore useful in hyperthyroidism, especially when other drugs are not tolerated. Colesevelam and ezetimibe have shown to improve glycemic control by reducing endogenous glucose production and enhancing glucagon-like polypeptide-1 (GLP-1) activity, respectively. Fenofibrate, a Peroxisome proliferator-activated receptor alpha (PPAR-α) agonist, is now known to prevent the progression of diabetic retinopathy by reducing oxidative stress but its role in diabetic neuropathy is yet to be proven in humans. Clofibrate, earlier used for partial central diabetes insipidus, enhances the release of arginine vasopressin (AVP) from the posterior pituitary. However, it is rarely used now with the ready availability of desmopressin. Statins have been tried in polycystic ovary disease for their ability to reduce testosterone levels, but they have failed to show any clinical benefit on ovulation rate. Statins are also associated with significant improvement in bone mineral density but did not lead to a reduction of fracture risk. Despite so many initial evidences, the use of lipid lowering agents in management of endocrinopathies is still in its infancy. We expect with better understanding of pathogenic mechanisms and further clinical outcome trials, lipid-lowering drugs will become an integral part of endocrine disorders.

INTRODUCTION

Lipid-lowering agents have effects beyond lipid-lowering and cardiovascular risk reduction. Indeed, they have been used in the treatment of endocrine conditions other than dyslipidemia. In this chapter, we discuss the clinical use of lipid-lowering agents in the management of a wide range of endocrine disorders. We discuss the role of fenofibrate and statins in diabetic retinopathy and neuropathy, cholestyramine in hyperthyroidism and colesevelam in glycemic control in diabetes. We also explore the use of clofibrate in diabetes insipidus, ezetimibe in diabetic dyslipidemia and the use statins in polycystic ovary syndrome (PCOS) and in improvement of bone health.

FENOFIBRATE IN DIABETIC RETINOPATHY

Fenofibrate is a PPAR-α (peroxisome proliferator-activated receptor alpha) agonist and it is typically used for the treatment of hypertriglyceridemia. In October 2013, Australia become the first country to approve the use of fenofibrate for the prevention of progression of diabetic retinopathy (DR). This approval was prompted by encouraging results from two significant randomized control trials, the FIELD study and the ACCORD-EYE study, both of which showed that fenofibrate significantly reduced the need for retinal laser therapy and reduced progression of DR.[1]

- *The FIELD study*: FIELD (Fenofibrate Intervention and Event Lowering in Diabetes) was a large prospective clinical trial comparing the impact of micronized fenofibrate versus placebo on the reduction of macrovascular and microvascular complications in a large cohort of patients with type 2 diabetes. Though fenofibrate did not show impressive results in terms of macrovascular risk reduction, it did show significant benefit in the need for laser photocoagulation therapy for maculopathy and proliferative DR.[1] There was a relative risk reduction in the need for laser therapy by 37% in the fenofibrate group over 5 years. The need for both first laser therapy and overall need for laser therapy was reduced in both patients with maculopathy and proliferative DR.[1] The FIELD study also analyzed the two-step progression of retinopathy grading as per ETDRS (Early Treatment Diabetic Retinopathy scale) in an ophthalmology sub-study, where sequential fundus photographs were taken at baseline, 2 years and 5 years. Among patients who did not have pre-existing DR at baseline, there was no significant reduction in two-step progression of retinopathy. However, for patients having pre-existing DR, there was a significant reduction in the same.[2]
- *ACCORD-EYE study*: The ACCORD lipid trial investigated the effect of adding fenofibrate to background simvastatin treatment and its impact on cardiovascular outcomes in individuals with type 2 diabetes. Addition of fenofibrate to simvastatin did not result in improved cardiovascular outcomes. In the ACCORD-EYE sub-study, the effect of fenofibrate on the progression of diabetic retinopathy was evaluated over a period of 4 years. In contrast to the FIELD study, these individuals had longer diabetes duration and higher background prevalence of DR. Both, intensive glycemic control and intensive control of dyslipidemia resulted in reduction in the progression of DR. In the intensive dyslipidemia control group, the progression of DR was compared among patients who received simvastatin plus fenofibrate versus those who received simvastatin plus placebo. Fenofibrate use resulted in a 40% reduction in progression of DR, defined as more than or equal to 3-step progression on the ETDRS scale or proliferative DR requiring laser or vitrectomy.[3] Benefits were more robust in those with pre-existing DR. The number needed to treat to prevent first laser treatment in FIELD study was 17 while the NNT to prevent progression of DR was 9 in the FIELD sub-study and 14 in the ACCORD-EYE study.[4]

Proposed Mechanism of Benefit in Retinopathy

Fenofibrate use is associated with significant reductions in triglycerides, modest reduction in total and low-density lipoprotein cholesterol (LDL-C) and elevation in apolipoprotein A1 (ApoA1) and high-density lipoprotein cholesterol. It also reduces small dense low-density lipoprotein (LDL) and remnant lipoproteins. However, the mechanism by which fenofibrate reduces DR is poorly understood. The postulated mechanisms include the following:

- Fenofibrate increases ApoA1 which is known to have a protective effective on DR. A recent study by Ankit et al. showed that mean ApoA1 has negative correlation with the severity of DR[5]
- Fenofibrate reduces intraretinal lipid transport and deposition and hence reduces lipotoxicity
- Fenofibrate acts primarily by suppressing PPAR-α, but also has anti-inflammatory and antiapoptotic effects. Nonlipid mechanisms of fenofibrate like reduction of apoptosis, angiogenesis and oxidative stress may be responsible for a reduced risk of DR.[1] Thus, it reduces retinal vascular permeability and suppresses the upregulation of collagen IV and fibronectin in the basal membrane of retinal capillaries. It also inhibits the apoptosis of retinal endothelial and retinal pigment epithelial cells. Its antioxidant effect also leads to increased nitric oxide mediated vasodilation in retinal arteries.

Apart from fenofibrate, statins and clofibrate have also been shown to have some benefit in DR, however robust evidence for the same is lacking. Statins are well known to reduce inflammation and curtail endothelial dysfunction. These effects could potentially prevent progression of diabetic retinopathy. Studies with various statins such as atorvastatin, pravastatin and simvastatin have shown mixed and inconsistent benefits.[6]

Clinical Pearl

Micronized fenofibrate in the dose of 200 mg/day can be used for prevention of progression of diabetic retinopathy and need for laser therapy amongst patients with pre-existing diabetic retinopathy.

CHOLESTYRAMINE IN HYPERTHYROIDISM

Cholesytramine is an anion exchange resin and bile acid sequestrant. It binds to components of bile which prevents its reabsorption in the gastrointestinal tract. It is indicated for use in dyslipidemia; however, it is also used off-label in the treatment of hyperthyroidism and in chronic diarrhea resulting from bile acid malabsorption.

While T4 and T3 are inactivated by deiodination, another important metabolic pathway includes the conjugation of the phenol hydroxyl group with glucuronic acid or sulfate. The glucuronides are rapidly excreted in bile but later hydrolyzed by bacterial β-glucouronidases in intestine. T3 and T4 are thus partly reabsorbed via enterohepatic circulation and partly excreted in feces. The enterohepatic circulation of T3 and T4 is increased in patients with hyperthyroidisim. Since cholesytramine binds to thyroid hormones in the intestine, it reduces their enterohepatic circulation and increases fecal excretion.[7]

SECTION 3: Management Issues in Lipocrinology

TABLE 1 Role of cholestyramine in Graves' disease

Indication	Dose
Graves' disease refractory to other medical management	1–2 g twice a day
Graves' disease in pregnancy refractory to other medications	1–2 g twice a day
Preoperative preparation for Graves' disease posted for thyroidectomy	2 g twice a day
Thyroid storm	4 g every 6 hours

In a randomized controlled trial (RCT), Kaykhaei et al. compared the use of cholestyramine plus methimazole plus propranolol versus placebo plus methimazole and propranolol in patients with Graves' disease. The authors found that addition of cholestyramine led to a greater and more rapid decline in thyroid hormone levels compared to placebo.[7]

Its use has been reported in individuals with iodinated contrast-induced and interferon-alpha (INF-α)-induced hyperthyroidism and thyroxine overdose related thyrotoxicosis. Cholestyramine can be considered for preoperative preparation of patients with Graves' disease if surgery is contemplated. This is particularly useful in cases where surgery is urgent. Cholestyramine can also be used for treatment of hyperthyroidism during pregnancy, especially in patients in whom thionamides are not tolerated or are contraindicated. It may also be useful as an adjuvant therapy in patients with thyroid storm, in the dose of 4 g every 6 hours. It is particularly useful in patients who are intolerant to or have contraindications to the use of thionamides.[8]

However, the clinical evidence for cholestyramine comes from case reports and it should not be considered as a front-line drug in the management of hyperthyroidism.

Clinical Pearl

The indications of cholestyramine in Graves' disease and the requisite doses have been tabulated in table 1.

CLOFIBRATE IN DIABETES INSIPIDUS

Clofibrate is typically used in the treatment of hypertriglyceridemia. It activates lipoprotein lipase and hence reduces very low-density lipoprotein levels. Clofibrate was withdrawn from the market in many countries since 2002 because of unexplained increase in mortality. One of the documented side effect of clofibrate is an increased risk of the syndrome of inappropriate antidiuretic hormone secretion and subsequent hyponatremia. The underlying mechanism driving this risk is not clear.[9]

Side effects of drugs have often been used for therapy. Clofibrate has been used for treatment of partial central diabetes insipidus where it was shown to significantly reduce free water clearance.[10] It has been observed that clofibrate only acts in patients who have some AVP reserve, hence it probably acts by enhancing the release of AVP from the posterior pituitary. Therefore, it cannot be used in patients with complete central diabetes insipidus. Additionally, it has not been found to be effective in patients with nephrogenic diabetes insipidus.[11] The evidence is limited to small case reports and case series in 1970s and subsequent use has declined since the ready availability of synthetic analogs of AVP, including DDAVP (desmopressin).

Apart from this, clofibrate has also been shown to help in the reduction of hard exudates in diabetic retinopathy but long-term clinical studies are lacking.

Clinical Pearl

Clofibrate in dose of 500 mg four times a day can be used in the treatment of partial central diabetes insipidus. However, poor availability of the drug combined with availability of better drugs for management of central diabetes insipidus has led to limited use of this agent in clinical practice.

STATINS IN POLYCYSTIC OVARY SYNDROME

Polycystic ovary syndrome is one of the most common endocrine conditions seen in women of reproductive age group. Hyperandrogenism combined with chronic oligo-anovulation are key clinical features of PCOS. In addition, PCOS is often associated with insulin resistance, dyslipidemia, chronic inflammation and endothelial dysfunction and a long-term increased cardiovascular risk.

A number of studies and subsequent meta-analysis have demonstrated that statins typically reduce testosterone in women with PCOS but have minimal effect on dihydroepiandrosterone sulfate (DHEA-S).[12] Higher testosterone levels are also associated with a more atherogenic lipid profile that is mitigated with the use of statins.[13] Several studies have demonstrated reduced LH levels with improvement in LH:FSH ratio with the use of statins. This is, in turn, associated with reduction in the size of the ovaries. Statins potentially reduce the chronic anovulation component of PCOS and hence may enhance fertility potential in these women.[13] In addition, they are potent lipid-lowering drugs and have other pleiotropic benefits, including immunomodulatory and anti-inflammatory properties and can provide ASCVD protection in women with PCOS. However, a Cochrane review concluded that despite improving the lipid parameters and reducing the testosterone levels, statins do not improve the clinical parameters in PCOS. Statins neither reduce the hirsutism and acne scores associated with PCOS, nor do they improve spontaneous ovulation and menstrual irregularity.[14]

In addition, there are significant concerns about the use of statins in this group of patients. Therefore, despite its potential benefits, use of statins in PCOS is still not popular. One of the major concerns pertains to an increased risk of new-onset diabetes with statin use. When statin is used primarily for cardiovascular risk reduction, their benefits far outweigh the risk of dysglycemia. However, women with PCOS are already at higher risk of development of diabetes. Hence, the risk benefit ratio of statins needs to be clearly ascertained in long term studies before they can be recommended.[13] Puurunen et al. reported that the use of statins in PCOS was associated with worsening of insulin resistance, thereby predisposing the patient to develop diabetes mellitus.[15] However, all statins do not seem to have similar effect on insulin resistance. While atorvastatin is associated with worsening of insulin resistance, pitavastain can potentially improve insulin sensitivity.[16] Pitavastatin was reported to have a favorable effect on glycemic control compared to atorvastatin in Japanese subjects.[17] It remains to be determined how statins would modify long-term cardiovascular risk in women with PCOS.

Another major concern is the risk of becoming pregnant while on statins. Polycystic ovary syndrome is a disease of reproductive age group. As it is mentioned above, statins can improve chronic anovulation in PCOS and hence there is a potential that these patients may have an unplanned pregnancy. Statins are contraindicated in pregnancy and have potential teratogenic effects, especially in early pregnancy.[13]

Clinical Pearl

It is premature at this point to consider the clinical use statins in PCOS, other than for management of dyslipidemia or in women with increased cardiovascular risk who are not planning pregnancy. Large RCTs are required to determine their role in PCOS. Pitvastatin shows promise in terms of improvement of insulin resistance; however, the evidence of the same is lacking at present.

STATINS FOR IMPROVEMENT OF BONE MINERAL DENSITY

Statins have demonstrated a positive effect on bone health with an increase in osteoblast differentiation and bone formation, related to the inhibition of isoprenoid biosynthetic pathway. They may also inhibit osteoclast differentiation and bone resorption by inhibiting the receptor activator of nuclear factor-κB (RANKL).

It has been suggested from number of observational studies that statins are associated with improvement of bone mineral density (BMD) and reduction of fracture risk. A meta-analysis published in 2016 concluded that the use of statins was associated with significant improvement in BMD but did not lead to a reduction in fracture risk.[18] An earlier meta-analysis had shown that despite observational studies showing beneficial effects of statins, RCTs have failed to show any significant benefit of statin in terms of either improvement of BMD or fracture prevention.[19]

The larger clinical trials for statin use like Scandinavian Simvastatin Survival Study (4S), Long-term Intervention with Pravastatin in Ischemic Disease (LIPID), and Heart Protection Study (HPS) have not shown any benefit of statin with regards to bone health.[20] It has been suggested that lipophilic statins like atorvastatin, lovastatin, and simvastatin are associated with better bone health parameters compared to hydrophilic statins like pravastatin, rosuvastatin, and fluvastatin.[21]

Clinical Pearl

The potential use of statins for bone health is an area of debate. At present the benefits of statins on bone health are ambiguous. The clinical use of statin for improvement of BMD or reduction of fracture risk is still premature based on current evidence.

EZETIMIBE IN DIABETES MELLITUS AND METABOLIC SYNDROME

In animal models, administration of ezetimibe was associated with reduction of dipeptidyl peptidase-4 (DPP4) activity and enhancement of glucagon-like polypeptide-1 (GLP1) levels. Hence, ezetimibe may have actions similar to DPP4 inhibitors.[22] In a meta-analysis, Wu and Wu have shown that the use of ezetimibe with low dose statin had a more favorable effect on glycemic parameters compared to high dose statins alone in patients with diabetes and dyslipidemia.[23] The IMPROVE-IT trial published in 2015 had demonstrated that the addition of ezetimibe to statins was associated with greater cardiovascular risk reduction compared to the use of statins alone in patients who had a recent acute coronary syndrome. A subgroup analysis showed that the benefit of ezetimibe was more in patients with diabetes compared to nondiabetics.[24] Yagi et al. demonstrated that in addition to LDL-C lowering, use of ezetimibe was associated with improvement in other parameters of metabolic syndrome such as reduction in urinary albumin excretion, reduction of insulin resistance and improvement in blood pressure.[25]

Clinical Pearl

The recent American Diabetes Association (ADA) guidelines have suggested that in patients with diabetes mellitus if the target LDL-C reduction is not achieved with the use of maximum tolerated dose of statins, the addition of ezetimibe is an effective option. Fixed dose combination of statin with 10 mg of ezetimibe is an effective option in patients with diabetes and dyslipidemia who do not tolerate high doses of statin.

FENOFIBRATE IN DIABETIC PERIPHERAL NEUROPATHY

Fibrates may have benefits in diabetic peripheral neuropathy (DPN) beyond their antiatherogenic effects in type 2 diabetes. The evidence of the effect of fenofibrate on DPN initially came from animal models. Cho et al.[26] showed fenofibrate exerts neuroprotective actions by ameliorating endothelial and/or nerve cell damage, at least in Schwann cells, and dampening inappropriate inflammatory responses in db/db mice. The beneficial effect was mediated by activation of PPAR-α, which attenuates or inhibits several vascular damage mediators, including inflammation, lipotoxicity, reactive oxygen species generation, endothelial dysfunction, and thrombosis. Recently, a small study by Davis et al.[27] showed that fibrate use was negatively associated (Odds ratio: 0.30, 95% CI 0.10–0.86; p = 0.025) with progression of DPN. However, similar results have not been replicated in larger trials.

Clinical Pearl

Unlike the use of fenofibrate for diabetic retinopathy, the use of fenofibrate for DPN still requires more evaluation before it can be recommended for routine clinical practice.

COLESEVELAM FOR TYPE 2 DIABETES MELLITUS

Bile acid sequestrants (BASs) (cholestyramine, colesevelam, colestilan, colestimide, and colestipol) are lipid-lowering agents for the treatment of hypercholesterolemia. These agents have been used either as monotherapy or in combination with statins, fibrates, and/or cholesterol absorption inhibitors for elevated LDL. Data from several studies suggest that in addition to significant lipid-lowering properties, BASs might also improve glycemic control in patients with type 2 diabetes. A study which was done for dyslipidemia in type 2 diabetes showed 13% reduction of plasma glucose after

6 weeks therapy with 8 g cholestyramine twice daily.[28] Colesevelam was evaluated in a large clinical trial program in adults with type 2 diabetes,[29] where it was shown to significantly improve glycemic control when added to existing glucose-lowering therapy in patients with type 2 diabetes.

Exact mechanism for its glycemic benefits is not known. Potential mechanisms include effects on the farnesoid X receptor (the bile acid receptor) in intestine and liver and TGR5 (a G protein-coupled receptor specific for bile acids) within the intestine, which may ultimately reduce endogenous glucose production.[30,31] Colesevelam is well tolerated when used throughout the type 2 diabetes continuum and can be used in combination with various anti-diabetes treatments. Incidence of hypoglycemia is low with colesevelam and its use was not associated with weight gain.[32]

Clinical Pearl

Colesevelam oral suspension in dose of 1.875 g orally twice a day can be a useful adjuvant in the management of type 2 diabetes. The absence of hypoglycemia and weight gain are additional benefits in diabetes mellitus.

CONCLUSION

The use of fenofibrate to prevent the progression of diabetic retinopathy, the use of cholestryramine in certain cases of hyperthyroidism and the use of ezetimibe and colesevelam for improved glycemic as well lipid management is substantiated by clinical evidence and may find merit in endocrinology practice. Meanwhile, the role of statins in bone health and PCOS management and the role of fenofibrate in neuropathy prevention needs further study. The use of clofibrate in partial central diabetes insipidus seems to be outdated with the easy availability of desmopressin in the modern era.

REFERENCES

1. Sharma N, Ooi JL, Ong J, et al. The use of fenofibrate in the management of patients with diabetic retinopathy: an evidence-based review. Aust Fam Physician. 2015;44(6):367-70.
2. Keech A, Mitchell P, Summanen P, et al. Effect of fenofibrate on the need for laser treatment for diabetic retinopathy (FIELD study): A randomised controlled trial. Lancet. 2007;370(9600):1687-97.
3. Chew EY, Ambrosius WT, Davis MD et al. Effects of medical therapies on retinopathy progression in type 2 diabetes. N Engl J Med. 2010;363(3):233-44.
4. Simó R, Ballarini S, Cunha-Vaz J, et al. Non-traditional systemic treatments for diabetic retinopathy: an evidence-based review. Curr Med Chem. 2015;22(21):2580-9.
5. Ankit BS, Mathur G, Agrawal RP, et al. Stronger relationship of serum apolipoprotein A-1 and B with diabetic retinopathy than traditional lipids. Indian J Endocrinol Metab. 2017;21(1):102-5.
6. Al-Janabi A, Lightman S, Tomkins-Netzer O. Statins in retinal disease. Eye (Lond). 2018;32(5):981-91.
7. Kaykhaei MA, Shams M, Sadegholvad A, et al. Low doses of cholestyramine in the treatment of hyperthyroidism. Endocrine. 2008;34(1-3):52-5.
8. Ross DS, Burch HB, Cooper DS, et al. 2016 American Thyroid Association guidelines for diagnosis and management of hyperthyroidism and other causes of thyrotoxicosis. Thyroid. 2016;26(10):1-272.
9. Oiso Y, Robertson GL, Nørgaard JP, Juul KV. Treatment of Neurohypophyseal diabetes insipidus. J Clin Endocrinol Metab. 2013;98(10):3958-67.

10. Kalra S, Zargar AH, Jain SM, et al. Diabetes insipidus: The other diabetes. Indian J Endocrinol Metab. 2016;20(1):9-21.
11. Bonnici F. Antidiuretic effect of clofibrate and carbamazepine in diabetes insipidus: studies on free water clearance and response to a water load. Clin Endocrinol (Oxf). 1973;2(3):265-75.
12. Gao L, Zhao FL, Li SC. Statin is a Reasonable Treatment Option for Patients with Polycystic Ovary Syndrome: a Meta-analysis of Randomized Controlled Trials. Exp Clin Endocrinol Diabetes. 2012;120(6):367-75.
13. Cassidy-Vu L, Joe E, Kirk JK. Role of statin drugs for polycystic ovary syndrome. J Fam Reprod Heal. 2016;10(4):165-75.
14. Raval AD, Hunter T, Stuckey B, Hart RJ. Statins for women with polycystic ovary syndrome not actively trying to conceive. Cochrane Database Syst Rev. 2011;(10):CD008565.
15. Puurunen J, Piltonen T, Puukka K, Ruokonen A, et al. Statin therapy worsens insulin sensitivity in women with polycystic ovary syndrome (PCOS): A prospective, randomized, double-blind, placebo-controlled study. J Clin Endocrinol Metab. 2013;98(12):4798-807.
16. Nakagomi A, Shibui T, Kohashi K, et al. Differential effects of atorvastatin and pitavastatin on inflammation, insulin resistance, and the carotid intima-media thickness in patients with dyslipidemia. J Atheroscler Thromb. 2015;22(11):1158-71.
17. Mita T, Nakayama S, Abe H, et al. Comparison of effects of pitavastatin and atorvastatin on glucose metabolism in type 2 diabetic patients with hypercholesterolemia. J Diabetes Investig. 2013;4(3):297-303.
18. Wang Z, Li Y, Zhou F, et al. Effects of statins on bone mineral density and fracture risk: A PRISMA-compliant systematic review and meta-analysis. Medicine (Baltimore). 2016;95(22):e3042.
19. Toh S, Hernández-Díaz S. Statins and fracture risk. A systematic review. Pharmacoepidemiol Drug Saf. 2007;16(6):627-40.
20. Rizzo M, Rini GB. Statins, fracture risk, and bone remodeling: What is true? Am J Med Sci. 2006332(2):55-60.
21. Luisetto G, Camozzi V. Statins, fracture risk, and bone remodeling. J Endocrinol Invest. 2009;32(4 Suppl):32-7.
22. Yang SJ, Choi JM, Kim L, et al. Chronic administration of ezetimibe increases active glucagon-like peptide-1 and improves glycemic control and pancreatic beta cell mass in a rat model of type 2 diabetes. Biochem Biophys Res Commun. 2011;407(1):153-7.
23. Wu H, Shang H, Wu J. Effect of ezetimibe on glycemic control: a systematic review and meta-analysis of randomized controlled trials. Endocrine. 2018;60(2):229-39.
24. Cannon CP, Blazing MA, Giugliano RP, et al. Ezetimibe added to statin therapy after acute coronary syndromes. N Engl J Med 2015;372(25):2387-97.
25. Yagi S, Akaike M, Aihara K, et al. Ezetimibe ameliorates metabolic disorders and microalbuminuria in patients with hypercholesterolemia. J Atheroscler Thromb. 2010;17(2):173-80.
26. Cho YR, Lim JH, Kim MY, et al. Therapeutic effects of fenofibrate on diabetic peripheral neuropathy by improving endothelial and neural survival in db/db mice. PLoS One. 2014;9(1):e83204.
27. Davis TM, Yeap BB, Davis WA, et al. Lipid-lowering therapy and peripheral sensory neuropathy in type 2 diabetes: the Fremantle diabetes study. Diabetologia. 2008;51(4):562-6.
28. Garg A, Grundy SM. Cholestyramine therapy for dyslipidemia in non-insulin-dependent diabetes mellitus: A short-term, double-blind, crossover trial. Ann Intern Med. 1994;121(6):416-22.
29. Fonseca VA, Rosenstock J, Wang AC, Truitt KE, Jones MR. Colesevelam HCl improves glycemic control and reduces LDL cholesterol in patients with inadequately controlled type 2 diabetes on sulfonylurea-based therapy. Diabetes Care. 2008;31(8):1479-84.
30. Goldfine AB. Modulating LDL cholesterol and glucose in patients with type 2 diabetes mellitus: targeting the bile acid pathway. Curr Opin Cardiol. 2008;23(5):502-11.
31. Staels B. A review of bile acid sequestrants: Potential mechanism (s) for glucose-lowering effects in type 2 diabetes mellitus. Postgrad Med. 2009;121(Suppl 1):25-30.
32. Handelsman Y. Role of bile acid sequestrants in the treatment of type 2 diabetes. Diabetes Care. 2011;34(Suppl 2):S244-50.

14
CHAPTER

Lipotropic Effects of Drugs Used in Endocrinology and Diabetes

Gagan Priya

ABSTRACT

Hormones are key regulators of adipose tissue distribution and function and have an important role in the regulation of lipid and lipoprotein metabolism. Hence, hormones used as replacement therapies in endocrine deficiency states and other drugs that alter endocrine function can have significant lipotropic effects. While some of these effects are beneficial to lipid health, others may be detrimental. For instance, thyroxine replacement in hypothyroid patients significantly improves dyslipidemia, while glucocorticoids have an unfavorable effect. In addition, diabetes is often associated with dyslipidemia and many antidiabetic agents influence lipids. In this chapter, we highlight the effects of various endocrine drugs on lipid physiology and lipid parameters to improve clinical decision making and patient care.

INTRODUCTION

Hormones are key regulators of adipose tissue distribution and function and have significant impact on lipid and lipoprotein metabolism. Therefore, it is important to understand the lipotropic effects of hormone-based and other endocrine therapies, as most of these therapies are required to be continued long-term and may affect the lipid health and cardiovascular (CV) risk of the individual. While some of these agents may have favorable effects on lipid fractions, others can adversely impact lipid health. In this chapter, we discuss the lipotropic effects of various hormone replacement therapies and medications used in diabetes management. These are summarized in table 1.

GROWTH HORMONE AXIS: LIPOTROPIC CONSIDERATIONS

Growth hormone (GH) increases the expression of hepatic low-density lipoprotein (LDL) receptors and increases LDL clearance. Additionally, it stimulates lipolysis and increases the availability of free fatty acids (FFAs) for triglyceride (TG) synthesis and very low-density lipoprotein (VLDL) production. Very low-density lipoprotein

CHAPTER 14: Lipotropic Effects of Drugs Used in Endocrinology and Diabetes

TABLE 1 Lipid effects of hormone-based therapies

Lipid parameter	Growth hormone	IGF-1	Thyroxine	Anti-thyroidal Drugs	Glucocorticoids	Testosterone	Androgen deprivation therapy	Estrogen	Estrogen and progesterone
Total cholesterol	Reduced	Reduced	Reduced	Increased	Increased	Decreased	Increased	Decreased	Decreased
LDL cholesterol	Reduced	Reduced	Reduced	Increased	No change/ Increased	Decreased	Increased	Decreased	Decreased
HDL cholesterol	No change/ increased	No change/ increased	No change/ reduced	No change	Increased	Decreased	Increased	Increased	Increased
Triglycerides	No change	No change	Reduced	No change	No change/ Increased	No change	Increased	Increased	Increased
Lipoprotein a	Increased	Reduced	Reduced	Increased	No change/ increased	Decreased	Increased	Decreased	Decreased

HDL, high-density lipoprotein; IGF-1, insulin-like growth factor 1; LDL, low-density lipoprotein.

secretion as well as clearance is increased, along with increased fatty acid oxidation. Growth hormone increases apolipoprotein A production, which leads to increased lipoprotein (a) [Lp (a)] levels.[1]

Growth Hormone Replacement Therapy

Adults with GH deficiency have increased visceral adiposity and elevated total cholesterol (TC), LDL cholesterol (LDL-C), and TGs along with reduced high-density lipoprotein cholesterol (HDL-C), leading to an increased CV risk. The effect of GH replacement therapy on serum lipids has been evaluated in several studies. Growth hormone treatment is associated with reduction in total cholesterol and LDL-C but has no effect HDL-C.[2] In some studies, however, GH was associated with increase in HDL-C.[2] Due to its lipolytic effect, the plasma non-esterified fatty acid (NEFA) concentration may be increased but TG levels are unaffected. The benefits of GH on LDL-C lowering are present over and above background use of statins.[3] Since GH acts via increasing LDL receptor expression, it has no effect on LDL-C levels in homozygous familial hypercholesterolemia, where functional LDL receptors are absent.[1] On the other hand, Lp (a) levels increase with GH treatment. Insulin-like growth factor 1 (IGF-1) treatment is associated with similar alterations in lipid levels, but the Lp (a) levels are reduced.[4] Discontinuation of GH therapy has been associated with worsening of lipid parameters in severe GH deficiency, Turner syndrome, and small-for-gestational-age children.[5] Growth hormone therapy reduces carotid intima media thickness (CIMT) in some but not all studies. Growth hormone replacement therapy has the potential to reduce CV risk in GH deficiency and this has been observed in few observational studies.[6] However, there is lack of long-term data from randomized controlled trials.

Treatment of Acromegaly

Acromegaly or GH excess is associated with increased TGs and low HDL-C. The effect of GH excess on TC and LDL-C is variable, but there is an increase in small dense LDL, apolipoprotein B (Apo B) and Lp (a). Treatment of acromegaly results in reduction in TGs and an increase in HDL-C levels.

PROLACTIN: LIPOTROPIC CONSIDERATIONS

Prolactin has been shown to reduce lipoprotein lipase activity, as has been seen in individuals with high prolactin levels due to prolactin-secreting pituitary adenomas. In addition, high prolactin suppresses estrogen secretion in women and may be associated with obesity. Therefore, individuals with prolactinomas have demonstrated elevated LDL-C and low HDL-C levels.

Dopamine Agonists

Dopamine agonists including cabergoline and bromocriptine are used for medical management of prolactinomas. They reduce total and LDL-C and may reduce TG levels. While some of these effects are believed to result from prolactin-lowering, dopamine agonists may possibly have an independent effect on lipid metabolism.[1]

THYROID: LIPOTROPIC CONSIDERATIONS

Thyroid hormones have widespread effects on lipid physiology. They induce cholesterol biosynthesis, by their effect on 3-hydroxy-3-methylglutaryl-coenzyme A (HMG-CoA) reductase. T3 also upregulates the LDL receptor gene expression, thereby increasing LDL clearance, both directly through thyroid hormone responsive elements (TREs) and indirectly through sterol regulatory element-binding protein-2 (SREBP-2).[7] However, the LDL lowering effect of thyroxine is seen even in the absence of LDL receptors (in LDL receptor knock-out mice).[1] T3 also reduces LDL oxidation, proprotein convertase subtilisin/kexin type 9 (PCSK9) activity, and Apo B synthesis.

Thyroid hormones increase the activity of cholesterol 7α-hydroxylase, resulting in increased conversion of cholesterol to bile acids. They also stimulate lipoprotein lipase (LPL) and hepatic lipase and increase cholesteryl ester transfer protein (CETP) activity, thereby affecting HDL metabolism and increasing reverse cholesterol transport. Through upregulation of apolipoprotein A5 (Apo A5), they reduce TG concentrations.[7] The effects of thyroid hormone on lipid metabolism are summarized in figure 1.

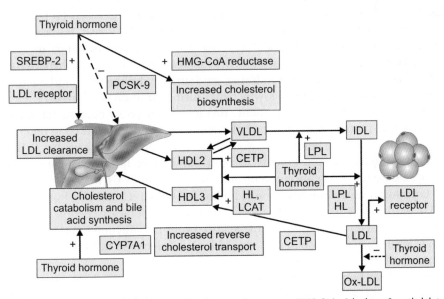

LDL, low-density lipoprotein; CETP, cholesteryl ester transfer protein; HMG-CoA, 3-hydroxy-3-methylglutaryl coenzyme A; VLDL, very low-density lipoprotein; IDL, intermediate-density lipoprotein; HDL, high-density lipoprotein; HL, hepatic lipase; LCAT, lecithin-cholesterol acyltransferase; Ox-LDL, oxidized low-density lipoprotein; PCSK9, proprotein convertase subtilisin/kexin type 9; SREBP-2, sterol regulatory element binding protein-2.

FIG. 1: Effect of thyroid hormones on lipoprotein metabolism. Thyroid hormone, particularly T3, acts via thyroid hormone responsive elements (TRE) on the promoter region of LDL receptor and upregulates its expression. In addition, it increases sterol regulatory element binding protein-2 (SREBP-2) which in turn increases LDL receptor expression. Thyroid hormones stimulate 7-alpha hydroxylase (CYP7A1), involved in cholesterol catabolism and increase bile acid synthesis. T3 upregulates HMG-CoA reductase and leads to increased cholesterol biosynthesis. CETP activity is increased, resulting in increased transport of cholesteryl esters from HDL2 to VLDL and IDL, thereby increasing reverse cholesterol transport. The hydrolysis of TG rich lipoproteins is stimulated by increase in lipoprotein lipase (LPL) activity. An increase in hepatic lipase mediates conversion of HDL2 to HDL3 and IDL to LDL. In addition, thyroid hormones also inhibit LDL oxidation.

Additionally, thyroid hormones affect adipocyte metabolism and production of adipokines. They regulate body weight, insulin sensitivity, oxidative stress, blood pressure, and endothelial and cardiac functions. Therefore, thyroid function assessment is recommended in individuals with dyslipidemia to exclude secondary dyslipidemia.

Thyroxine Replacement Therapy

There exists a linear relationship between thyroid-stimulating hormone (TSH) concentration and TC, LDL-C, and TGs and an inverse relationship with HDL-C, even within the normal range of TSH. Both overt and subclinical hypothyroidism (SCH) is associated with increased TC and LDL-C, modestly increased TG and VLDL, and increased Lp (a) concentrations. Even though HMG-CoA reductase activity is reduced, there is reduced LDL and intermediate-density lipoprotein (IDL) clearance, resulting from reduced LDL receptor activity. In addition, LPL activity is reduced which leads to a reduced clearance of TG-rich lipoproteins. High-density lipoprotein cholesterol levels may be elevated due to increased concentration of HDL2 particles and reduced activity of CETP in overt hypothyroidism, but reduced HDL-C has been observed in SCH. Hypothyroidism is also associated with increased Lp (a) levels.[8] While overt hypothyroidism is associated with increased CV risk, the association of SCH and dyslipidemia remains disputed with conflicting evidence in several studies. Hypothyroidism is associated with increased body weight, hypertension, insulin resistance, metabolic syndrome, endothelial dysfunction, and increased homocysteine and uric acid levels, which may further attribute to CV risk.

Levothyroxine (LT4) replacement therapy in hypothyroidism significantly improves lipid metabolism. In fact, cholesterol levels were considered to determine adequacy of treatment before the availability of radioimmunoassays for TSH and thyroid hormones.[1] Improvements in lipid parameters have been correlated to improvements in free T4 concentration and can occur within 4–6 weeks of initiation of LT4. Levothyroxine therapy results in reduction in TC, LDL-C, and TGs, but no change in LDL particle size has been observed.[9] Greater reductions are seen in individuals with higher baseline TSH. Levothyroxine also results in reduction in Lp (a) and TGs. HDL-C levels may decrease in some individuals.[8] A decrease in CIMT with LT4 has been observed in some studies.[7]

Inconsistent benefits of LT4 substitution therapy on lipids have been seen in individuals with SCH. While some studies demonstrated reduction in TC, LDL-C, and Lp (a), reduced CIMT, and improved endothelial function, this has not been replicated in other studies.[9] Individuals with TSH more than 10 mIU/L, higher initial cholesterol levels, and thyroid autoimmunity are more likely to benefit from LT4.[7] However, if lipid parameters do not improve with adequate LT4 replacement, primary dyslipidemia should be considered and lipid-lowering therapy initiated.

Thyromimetics

Development of thyroid hormone analogs began in 1980s. Dextrothyroxine (D-enantiomer of thyroxine) was found to have a positive effect on LDL-C levels but increased CV mortality. The effect of thyroid hormones on lipid metabolism is primarily mediated through thyroid hormone receptor TRβ, while extrahepatic effects are mediated through TRα. This has generated interest in development of thyromimetics that are liver-selective and TRβ-specific, as potential lipid-lowering agents. These include sobetirome, eprotirome, MB07811, and MGL3196. Thyromimetics are aimed to increase basal metabolic rate, promote weight loss and cholesterol reduction, while avoiding side-effects such as tachycardia, bone loss or hypothalamic-pituitary-thyroid (HPT) axis suppression.[10] The lipid-lowering effect of thyromimetics is attributed to increased hepatic LDL clearance, reduced expression of SREBP-1c, and increased expression of HDL receptor SR-B1 (reverse cholesterol transport). Initial studies reported that eprotirome reduced cholesterol as well as Lp (a) levels. But in a phase III trial, it displayed a significant potential to induce liver injury and further development of this molecule was abandoned.[10] While TRβ agonists may hold promise in the management of dyslipidemia, there are significant challenges in designing tissue-specific and receptor-selective compounds and most agents have not progressed to phase III trials.

Treatment of Hyperthyroidism

Individuals with hyperthyroidism have lower levels of TC, LDL-C, and Lp (a) and lower HDL-C, while TGs remain unchanged. Hyperthyroidism leads to a decrease in PCSK9 activity and can be a cause of acquired hypobetalipoproteinemia. Treatment of hyperthyroidism with antithyroidal drugs restores these alterations in lipid parameters.

GLUCOCORTICOIDS: LIPOTROPIC CONSIDERATIONS

Glucocorticoids increase the availability of substrate (glucose, amino acids, and fatty acids) for mitochondrial oxidation by increasing lipolysis, gluconeogenesis, and proteolysis. They influence adipose tissue biology in several aspects by their effect on adipogenesis, lipid metabolism, inflammation, and adipokine production.[11] In the liver, glucocorticoids increase the activity of acetyl-CoA carboxylase and fatty acid synthase and stimulate fatty acid synthesis. They also stimulate enzymes involved in TG synthesis. The increase in hepatic TG synthesis leads to decreased degradation of Apo B, increased synthesis and secretion of VLDL, and increased LDL-C levels.[12] In adipose tissue, glucocorticoids increase the hydrolysis of circulating TGs (chylomicrons and VLDL) by increasing LPL activity, the effect being more prominent in omental than subcutaneous adipose tissue. They also increase cyclic adenosine monophosphate (cAMP) levels, which stimulate the activation of protein kinase A (PKA) leading to phosphorylation of hormone-sensitive lipase. By these mechanisms, there is increase in circulating FFA concentration.[13] This promotes ectopic fat deposition in liver, muscle and visceral adipose tissue, and adipose tissue hypertrophy. Glucocorticoids also increase the conversion of preadipocytes to mature adipocytes, with resultant adipose tissue hyperplasia. Central fat depots are more responsive to glucocorticoids. In addition, Apo A1 secretion and lecithin–cholesterol acyltransferase (LCAT) activity is increased and hepatic lipase activity decreased, resulting in increase in HDL cholesterol.

The effect on lipid metabolism is mediated through glucocorticoid receptors (GR). While glucocorticoids reduce the expression of proinflammatory cytokines (interleukin-6 and plasminogen activator inhibitor 1) through their effect on GR, their action via mineralocorticoid receptor (MR) results in increased expression of proinflammatory cytokines.

Glucocorticoid Therapy

Glucocorticoid therapy has variable effects on lipid parameters, depending on the dose being used (physiological or supra-physiological), route of administration (topical or systemic), and the underlying disease for which they are administered and concomitant medications.[14] High-dose glucocorticoids acutely increase systemic lipolysis and increase FFA levels, while long-term administration promotes central fat deposition.[11] Low doses seem to have minimal effect on lipids, while high doses are associated with increased TGs, LDL-C, and HDL-C. Long-term oral glucocorticoid use has been associated with increased CV risk, which is higher with greater dose, longer exposure, and current use.[13]

No significant change in plasma lipids has been demonstrated with inhaled or topical steroids. In noninflammatory states, there is an increase in HDL-C with variable effect on LDL-C and TGs. In inflammatory conditions, the anti-inflammatory effect of glucocorticoids confounds their direct effect on lipid metabolism. In post-transplant patients, the effect of glucocorticoids is difficult to segregate from other immunosuppressants being administered. Dexamethasone, which is a selective GR agonist, decreases proinflammatory cytokine expression in adipose tissue.[11]

11β-hydroxysteroid dehydrogenase type 1 (11β-HSD1) regulates the conversion of inactive cortisone to active cortisol in adipose tissue. 11β-hydroxysteroid dehydrogenase type 1 inhibitors are under development as potential therapeutic options for treatment for obesity and diabetes. While they improve insulin sensitivity, they also limit glucocorticoid-induced lipolysis and decrease TC, FFA, and TG levels. Compensatory upregulation of hypothalamic-pituitary-adrenal (HPA) axis with resultant adrenal hypertrophy and effects on immune system has limited development of these drugs.

Medical Management of Cushing Syndrome

Central obesity and insulin resistance is a characteristic feature of endogenous hypercortisolism or Cushing syndrome and contributes to lipid abnormalities and hyperglycemia. Dyslipidemia with increased TC, LDL-C, TGs, and VLDL is common in patients with Cushing syndrome and correlates with disease severity. The effect on Lp (a) and HDL-C is variable.[1] Overall, the risk of CVD is increased.

Treatment of Cushing syndrome results in significant improvement in hyperlipidemia and reduces CV risk. Ketoconazole blocks several steps in cholesterol biosynthesis and reduces TC, IDL-C, LDL-C, and Apo B levels. For these reasons, it was used in the treatment of familial hypercholesterolemia before the availability of statins. However, it inhibits several hepatic P450 enzymes. Thus, it may increase the risk of myotoxicity with statins metabolized by cytochrome P450 CYP3A4, including simvastatin, atorvastatin, and lovastatin.[1] Mitotane inhibits steroidogenesis and increases circulating levels of cortisol, LDL-C, and Apo B, while the effect on TGs, HDL-C, and Lp (a) is variable.

DIABETES MEDICATIONS: LIPOTROPIC CONSIDERATIONS

Diabetes and metabolic syndrome are associated with increased visceral and ectopic fat deposition, insulin resistance, and increased FFA secretion. The typical lipid abnormalities seen in diabetes include reduced HDL-C, elevated TGs, and elevated small dense LDL-C, referred to as atherogenic dyslipidemia. Both fasting and postprandial TG-rich lipoproteins (VLDL, IDL, and chylomicrons) are increased and there is an overproduction of Apo B-48 and Apo B-100, along with abnormal lipolysis. This is associated with significantly increased risk of CV disease and mortality and therefore, the effects of various antidiabetic medications on lipid parameters and CV risk is of immense interest.

Metformin

Metformin is considered as the first-choice drug for the management of type 2 diabetes due to its good efficacy and tolerability, low-risk of hypoglycemia, long-term safety, pleiotropic benefits, and cardioprotective potential. Metformin acts via inhibition of the mitochondrial respiratory chain, creating a state of cellular energy deficit. Subsequent activation of cellular 5′ adenosine monophosphate-activated protein kinase (AMPK) leads to increased glucose uptake and utilization and increased β-oxidation of fatty acids, along with downregulation of metabolic pathways that consume energy, including gluconeogenesis, lipid and protein synthesis, and cell proliferation. Metformin leads to reduction in visceral fat, though overall effect on body weight is considered as neutral. It leads to small but significant reductions in LDL-C and TC with slight reduction in TG and trend toward increase in HDL-C.[15]

Thiazolidinediones

Thiazolidinediones act as agonists for peroxisome proliferator-activated receptor gamma (PPAR-γ) and improve insulin sensitivity. They also have anti-inflammatory, anti-oxidant, and anti-proliferative effects. Pioglitazone differs from rosiglitazone in the genes activated downstream of PPAR-γ signaling and is also a partial activator of PPAR-α. Though pioglitazone leads to expansion of adipocyte mass and an increase in body weight and BMI, this is not associated with a negative metabolic profile. Rather, pioglitazone results in increased differentiation of preadipocytes to insulin-sensitive mature adipocytes and a redistribution of fat from visceral to subcutaneous fat depots. This results in improved insulin sensitivity and reduced lipotoxicity and confers pioglitazone with hepatoprotective and cardioprotective properties.[16] There is a significant reduction in TGs and increase in HDL-C. Although there is a small increase in TC and LDL-C, the TC to HDL ratio decreases and the LDL particle size increases, making it less atherogenic.[14] In long-term trials, pioglitazone has demonstrated cardioprotective effects in diabetic and prediabetic individuals, though it increases the risk for heart failure. However, similar beneficial effects on lipid profile are not seen with rosiglitazone, which has been associated with increased CV risk.

In contrast to pioglitazone, rosiglitazone increases TG levels, causes a smaller increase in HDL-C, and a greater increase in LDL-C. Saroglitazar, a dual PPAR-α/γ agonist with predominant PPAR-α activity results in significant reduction in TGs with modest reductions in glycemia. However, long-term studies are lacking.

Glucagon-like Peptide-1 Receptor Agonists

Glucagon-like peptide-1 (GLP-1) receptor agonists (RAs) stimulate insulin production and inhibit glucagon secretion, reduce hyperglycemia, delay gastric emptying, promote satiety, and reduce abdominal obesity and body weight. Glucagon-like peptide-1 RAs reduce postprandial rise in TGs and FFAs and lead to improvement in fasting as well as postprandial lipid levels. Glucagon-like peptide-1 receptor signaling modulates key enzymes of lipid metabolism in the liver, reduces hepatic TG content, reduces production of TGs and VLDL from the liver, and impairs *de novo* lipogenesis and β-oxidation. It also modulates reverse cholesterol transport.[17] Exenatide treatment was associated with lower TG, Apo B-48, Apo C-III, and NEFA levels following high-calorie, high-fat diet up to 8 hours postprandially.[14] They lead to modest reductions in LDL-C, TC, and TGs, but the effect on HDL-C is not significant.[17] The effect on lipid parameters is independent of their glucose-lowering and weight-reducing effect. Glucagon-like peptide-1 RAs have additional anti-atherogenic properties because they reduce the expression of inflammatory mediators, suppress smooth muscle cell proliferation, and stimulate nitric oxide production. They may have direct myocardial effects as well. Indeed, liraglutide demonstrated reduction in CV outcomes in the LEADER trial.

Dipeptidyl Peptidase-4 Inhibitors

Dipeptidyl peptidase-4 (DDP-4) inhibitors reduce the breakdown of endogenous GLP-1. There is limited data on the effect of DPP-4 inhibitors on lipid parameters. Vildagliptin improved postprandial TG and Apo B-48-containing TG-rich lipoprotein particle metabolism after high fat diet.[14] Similar improvements in postprandial lipemia have been reported with sitagliptin.[17] Sitagliptin was associated with a small but significant decrease in TC and TGs and a small increase in HDL-C, but no effect on LDL-C. Dipeptidyl peptidase-4 inhibitors have a neutral effect on CV risk, though saxagliptin and alogliptin are associated with increased risk of hospitalization for heart failure.

Sodium-glucose Co-transporter 2 Inhibitors

Sodium-glucose co-transporter 2 inhibitors reduce renal glucose reabsorption and cause urinary glucose loss, contributing to their glucose-lowering effect. In addition, they also promote natriuresis. These effects lead to significant reduction in blood pressure and body weight with greater reduction in fat mass than lean body mass. Sodium-glucose co-transporter 2 inhibitors lead to a modest but statistically significant increase in HDL-C and slight increase in LDL-C and TC, with no change in LDL/HDL ratio or TGs.[18] Sodium-glucose co-transporter 2 inhibitors, particularly empagliflozin, have demonstrated significant cardioprotective properties independent of their glycemic and lipid effects.

Alpha-glucosidase Inhibitors

Alpha-glucosidase inhibitors (AGIs) delay intestinal carbohydrate absorption and reduce postprandial glucose and TG excursions and decrease Apo C-III. Thus, they improve postprandial hyperlipidemia in addition to their effect on postprandial hyperglycemia. In randomized trials, acarbose demonstrated significant reduction in TGs and VLDL and an increase in HDL-C, while LDL-C and TC remain unaffected.[19] However, their ability to reduce postprandial hyperlipidemia is of greater interest in their potential cardioprotective effects.

Sulfonylureas

Sulfonylureas are potent glucose-lowering agents but are limited by an increased risk of hypoglycemia and weight gain. Previous studies inconsistently reported a negative effect of sulfonylureas on lipid metabolism. In a recent meta-analysis, second and third generation sulfonylureas were found to increase the levels of FFAs and TGs and decrease HDL-C and LDL-C, with no effect on TC, Apo A1, or Apo B.[20] The overall effect on lipids seems to be minimal.

Insulin

In addition to its effect on glucose metabolism, insulin plays a key role in lipid, protein, and nucleic acid metabolism. Insulin stimulates adipose tissue LPL, resulting in increased clearance of chylomicrons and VLDL particles from circulation.[14] Fatty acid delivery to adipose tissue is increased with increased TG synthesis in adipocytes. LPL activity in skeletal muscle is reduced, thus reducing a tendency for myocellular fat deposition. It inhibits hormone-sensitive lipase in adipocytes and reduces lipolysis.[1] Therefore, insulin reduces circulating TGs and TG-rich lipoproteins, ameliorating key defects in atherogenic dyslipidemia. Acute increase in insulin promotes LDL clearance by increase LDL receptor expression. Additionally, insulin has potent vasodilatory, anti-inflammatory, antiplatelet, and antiatherogenic properties.

ANDROGENS: LIPOTROPIC CONSIDERATIONS

Testosterone upregulates two genes involved in the catabolism of HDL-C, hepatic lipase, and scavenger receptor B1 (SR-B1). Scavenger receptor B1 further increases uptake of cholesterol into steroidogenic cells and hepatocytes and increases cholesterol efflux from peripheral cells. Hepatic lipase further facilitates the action of SR-B1 by hydrolyzing phospholipids on the surface of HDL particles, thus decreasing HDL particle size, releasing Apo A1 and increasing the degradation of Apo A1.[21] These changes result in reduction of HDL-C. Testosterone antagonizes the effect of estrogen to stimulate LDL receptor expression and may result in increased LDL-C. It also reduces Lp (a) through undefined mechanisms.

Testosterone affects body fat composition and muscle mass and testosterone deficient males have increased visceral adiposity and impaired insulin sensitivity.[22] Low testosterone levels in men are associated with a proatherogenic lipid pattern, with low HDL cholesterol and Apo A1 and increased TC, LDL-C, Apo B, and TGs and trend toward increased Lp (a) levels.[21] Cross-sectional studies suggest an increased CV risk in hypogonadal men, but this has not been established in prospective long-term studies.

Testosterone Replacement Therapy

Testosterone replacement therapy leads to reduced body fat mass, especially central adiposity, and improved insulin sensitivity. The changes in lipid parameters have been variable. Factors that influence these differences include the dose and type of testosterone preparation, whether it can be aromatized to estrogens, route of administration, and duration of treatment and underlying indication for use.[1] Intramuscular testosterone treatment was associated with reduction in body fat and increase in muscle mass, along with a reduction in TC and LDL-C even in patients on statins, but a reduction in HDL-C and an insignificant change in TGs.[22] Transdermal testosterone preparations have a lesser effect on HDL-C while high-dose testosterone lowers HDL-C more significantly. Testosterone administration also decreases Lp (a) concentrations.[23] The effects of testosterone on lipids may be counterbalanced by aromatization to estrogen that increases HDL-C and decreases LDL-C. Testosterone preparations that do not get aromatized to estrogen are associated with more significant reductions in HDL-C and LDL-C.

When used in physiological replacement doses in hypogonadal men, the relative effect on lipid parameters is minimal. Moreover, in observational and randomized trials of testosterone treatment in older men, no significant CV effects have been reported. But high-dose, more potent androgen therapy, used for increasing muscle mass and muscle strength in young men, such as nandrolone-decanoate or oxandrolone that do not get aromatized, can have significant impact with marked reduction in HDL-C and increase in LDL-C.[1] Simultaneous use of aromatase inhibitors further compounds these effects. The finding of an unexpectedly low HDL-C in an athletic male should prompt suspicion about the use of androgens or anabolic steroids.

Androgen Deprivation Therapy

Androgen deprivation therapy (orchidectomy or GnRH antagonists in patients with prostate cancer) increases LDL-C, Lp (a), and TG levels. But HDL-C and Apo A1 concentrations increase within weeks of lowering testosterone levels, in contrast to the relationship of serum testosterone with HDL-C in hypogonadal states. Androgen deprivation therapies have been associated with increased CV risk and mortality.[1]

Dehydroepiandrosterone Supplementation

Dehydroepiandrosterone (DHEA) has often been promoted for use in patients with hypoadrenalism and in elderly men and postmenopausal women for its proposed benefits in metabolic and skeletomuscular health, with little evidence to support its use. The action of DHEA is mediated primarily via conversion to sex steroids that modulate adipose tissue and muscle mass and insulin sensitivity. Studies have failed to demonstrate any positive effect of DHEA on insulin sensitivity, body weight, and adiposity or lipids in elderly men and women.[24] In women with hypoadrenalism,

DHEA supplementation had an unfavorable effect on lipid parameters with significant reductions seen in HDL-C and slight decrease in LDL-C and TGs.[25]

ESTROGEN AND PROGESTERONE: LIPOTROPIC CONSIDERATIONS

Estrogen increases the synthesis of Apo A1, that leads to increased formation of HDL. By inhibiting the expression of SR-B1 and hepatic lipase and thereby, reducing the hydrolysis of TGs and phospholipids on HDL particles, it decreases the catabolism of HDL. Estrogen also increases the hepatic expression of LDL receptors and increases LDL clearance. It also reduces PCSK9 levels and reduces the degradation of LDL receptors, which further contributes to LDL reduction. However, the production and secretion of VLDL particles is increased, resulting in an increase in TGs.[1]

Progestins can act via the androgen receptor and the effect of various progestins on lipids depends on their androgenic potential. Progesterone results in a decrease in HDL-C and TGs but has no effect on Lp (a) levels and a minimal effect on LDL-C. More androgenic progestins, such as norgestrel and norethindrone acetate, are likely to have greater effects on lipids.

The HDL-C levels are relatively higher and LDL-C and TG levels lower in pre-menopausal women, compared to men.[1] Following menopause, there is an increase in total and central adiposity along with an increase in LDL-C and Lp (a) levels with small decrease in HDL-C.

Estrogen Treatment

Estrogen therapy, including conjugated estrogens and estradiol, is related with a rise in HDL-C and TGs and decrease in LDL-C and Lp (a). Estrogen can cause marked increase in TGs in patients at risk of hypertriglyceridemia. The effect of transdermal preparations on lipid fractions, however, is less robust as it bypasses first-pass hepatic metabolism and it should be preferred over oral formulations in patients with hypertriglyceridemia.[26] The selective estrogen receptor modulator, tamoxifen, has been shown to reduce TC, LDL-C, and Lp (a) with an increase in TGs but no significant change in HDL-C.[27]

Estrogen and Progesterone

In combined oral contraceptive pills, progesterone blunts the estrogen-mediated rise in HDL-C but has no effect on LDL-C, which reduces due to the estrogen component. Compared to statins, combined oral contraceptives cause smaller reductions in LDL-C, more marked reductions in Lp (a), similar increase in HDL-C but a rise in TGs. The effect of hormone replacement therapy (HRT) is variable and affected by type of estrogen and progesterone used, dosing, route of administration, baseline lipid levels, and underlying metabolic abnormalities.

While HRT in postmenopausal women has been associated with lower CV risk in observational studies, the same has not been observed in large randomized clinical trials.[28] Rather, adverse CV signal was noted in the Women's Health Initiative, especially in elderly women and those with underlying CV risk factors.[29] Oral contraceptives with higher estrogen doses (>50 µg) likely increase CV risk.[30]

In addition, HRT is associated with an increased risk of thromboembolic events. Therefore, HRT is not recommended for CV risk reduction and should only be used for refractory postmenopausal symptoms for short-term.

CONCLUSION

Several endocrine disorders are associated with lipid alterations that are partly amenable to treatment of underlying disease. Key drugs used in endocrine disease states have variable effects on lipid profile. While some of these endocrine drugs such as growth hormone preparations, levothyroxine, estrogen, metformin, piolitazone, etc., have beneficial effects on lipids, other drugs such as glucocorticoids, anabolic steroids, rosiglitazone, etc. may have detrimental effects. An understanding of these lipotropic effects is important in the decision-making process when treating endocrine disorders.

REFERENCES

1. Feingold K, Brinton EA, Grunfeld C. The effect of endocrine disorders on lipids and lipoproteins. In: De Groot LJ, Chrousos G, Dungan K, Feingold KR, Grossman A, Hershman JM, Koch C, Korbonits M, McLachlan R, New M, Purnell J, Rebar R, Singer F, Vinik A (Eds). Endotext [Internet]. South Dartmouth (MA): MDText.com, Inc.; 2000-2017.
2. Newman CB, Carmichael JD, Kleinberg DL. Effects of low dose versus high dose human growth hormone on body composition and lipids in adults with GH deficiency: a meta-analysis of placebo-controlled randomized trials. Pituitary. 2015;18(3):297-305.
3. Monson JP, Jönsson P, Koltowska-Häggström M, et al. Growth hormone (GH) replacement decreases serum total and LDL-cholesterol in hypopituitary patients on maintenance HMG CoA reductase inhibitor (statin) therapy. Clin Endocrinol (Oxf). 2007;67(4):623-8.
4. Olivecrona H, Johansson AG, Lindh E, et al. Hormonal regulation of serum lipoprotein(a) levels. Contrasting effects of growth hormone and insulin-like growth factor-I. Arterioscler Thromb Vasc Biol. 1995;15(7):847-9.
5. Rothermel J, Lass N, Bosse C, et al. Impact of discontinuation of growth hormone treatment on lipids and weight status in adolescents. J Pediatr Endocrinol Metab. 2017;30(7):749-57.
6. van Bunderen CC, van Nieuwpoort IC, Arwert LI, et al. Does growth hormone replacement therapy reduce mortality in adults with growth hormone deficiency? Data from the Dutch National Registry of Growth Hormone Treatment in adults. J Clin Endocrinol Metab. 2011;96(10):3151-9.
7. Rizos C, Elisaf M, Liberopoulos E. Effects of thyroid dysfunction on lipid profile. Open Cardiovasc Med J. 2011;5:76-84.
8. Duntas LH, Brenta G. The effect of thyroid disorders on lipid levels and metabolism. Med Clin North Am. 2012;96(2):269-81.
9. Asranna A, Taneja RS, Kulshreshta B. Dyslipidemia in subclinical hypothyroidism and the effect of thyroxine on lipid profile. Indian Endocrinol Metab. 2012;16(Suppl 2):S347-9.
10. Jakobsson T, Vedin LL, Parini P. Potential role of thyroid receptor β agonists in the treatment of hyperlipidemia. Drugs. 2017;77(15):1613-21.
11. Lee MJ, Pramyothin P, Karastergiou K, et al. Deconstructing the roles of glucocorticoids in adipose tissue biology and the development of central obesity. Biochim Biophys Acta. 2014;1842(3):473-81.
12. Peckett AJ, Wright DC, Riddell MC. The effects of glucocorticoids on adipose tissue lipid metabolism. Metabolism. 2011;60(11):1500-10.
13. Geer EB, Islam J, Buettner C. Mechanisms of glucocorticoid-induced insulin resistance: focus on adipose tissue function and lipid metabolism. Endocrinol Metab Clin North Am. 2014;43(1):75-102.
14. Mihailescu DV, Vora A, Mazzone T. Lipid effects of endocrine medications. Curr Atheroscler Rep. 2011;13(1):88-94.

15. Wulffelé MG, Kooy A, de Zeeuw D, et al. The effect of metformin on blood pressure, plasma cholesterol and triglycerides in type 2 diabetes mellitus: a systematic review. J Intern Med. 2004;256(1):1-14.
16. Filipova E, Uzunova K, Kalinov K, et al. Effects of pioglitazone therapy on blood parameters, weight and BMI: a meta-analysis. Diabetol Metab Syndr. 2017;9:90.
17. Zhong J, Maiseyeu A, Rajagopalan S. Lipoprotein effects of incretin analogs and dipeptidyl peptidase 4 inhibitors. Clin Lipidol. 2015;10(1):103-12.
18. Yanai H, Katsuyama H, Hamasaki H, et al. Sodium-Glucose Cotransporter 2 Inhibitors: Possible Anti-Atherosclerotic Effects Beyond Glucose Lowering. J Clin Med Res. 2016;8(1):10-4.
19. Monami M, Vitale V, Ambrosio ML, et al. Effects on lipid profile of dipeptidyl peptidase 4 inhibitors, pioglitazone, acarbose, and sulfonylureas: meta-analysis of placebo-controlled trials. Adv Ther. 2012;29(9):736-46.
20. Chen YH, Du L, Geng XY, et al. Effects of sulfonylureas on lipids in type 2 diabetes mellitus: a meta-analysis of randomized controlled trials. J Evid Based Med. 2015;8(3):134-48.
21. Vodo S, Bechi N, Petroni A, et al. Testosterone-induced effects on lipids and inflammation. Mediators Inflamm. 2013;2013:183041.
22. Kelly DM, Jones TH. Testosterone: a metabolic hormone in health and disease. J Endocrinol. 2013;217(3):R25-45.
23. Cai X, Tian Y, Wu T, et al. Metabolic effects of testosterone replacement therapy on hypogonadal men with type 2 diabetes mellitus: a systematic review and meta-analysis of randomized controlled trials. Asian J Androl. 2014;16(1):146-52.
24. Elraiyah T, Sonbol MB, Wang Z, et al. Clinical review: The benefits and harms of systemic dehydroepiandrosterone (DHEA) in postmenopausal women with normal adrenal function: a systematic review and meta-analysis. J Clin Endocrinol Metab. 2014;99(10):3536-42.
25. Srinivasan M, Irving BA, Dhatariya K, et al. Effect of dehydroepiandrosterone replacement on lipoprotein profile in hypoadrenal women. J Clin Endocrinol Metab. 2009;94(3):761-4.
26. Goodman MP. Are all estrogens created equal? A review of oral vs. transdermal therapy. J Womens Health (Larchmt). 2012;21(2):161-9.
27. Love RR, Wiebe DA, Feyzi JM, et al. Effects of tamoxifen on cardiovascular risk factors in postmenopausal women after 5 years of treatment. J Natl Cancer Inst. 1994;86(20):1534-9.
28. Manson JE, Chlebowski RT, Stefanick ML, et al. Menopausal hormone therapy and health outcomes during the intervention and extended poststopping phases of the Women's Health Initiative randomized trials. JAMA. 2013;310(13):1353-68.
29. Manson JE, Hsia J, Johnson KC, et al. Estrogen plus progestin and the risk of coronary heart disease. N Engl J Med. 2003;349(6):523-34.
30. Roach RE, Helmerhorst FM, Lijfering WM, et al. Combined oral contraceptives: the risk of myocardial infarction and ischemic stroke. Cochrane Database Syst Rev. 2015;(8):CD011054.

CHAPTER 15

Endocrine Effects of Lipid-lowering Drugs

Yashpal Singh

ABSTRACT

Lipid-lowering drugs are among the most widely prescribed drugs and have a significant role in the secondary as well as primary prevention of cardiovascular disease. Most of these drugs have pleiotropic effects, including a myriad of endocrine effects as well. Statins affect glucose metabolism by affecting both insulin secretion and insulin sensitivity and their use has been associated with an increased risk of new onset diabetes. On the other hand, drugs such as colesevelam have a favorable effect on glucose profile. Statins increase the risk of myopathy, especially in patients at high risk of muscle-related symptoms and those using concomitant drugs such as fibrates. They have been shown to have a positive effect on bone health and act by increasing bone formation and reducing bone resorption. A beneficial effect on erectile dysfunction in men and hyperandrogenemia in polycystic ovary syndrome (PCOS) has also been reported. The bile acid sequestrant cholestyramine increases fecal excretion of thyroid hormones and has been used as an adjunctive treatment in hyperthyroidism. Clinicians are often faced with the challenge of identifying a therapeutic regimen that achieves the desired lipid goals but is well tolerated by the patient. In this chapter, the authors elaborate on the available evidence on endocrine effects of lipid-lowering drugs and their clinical implications.

INTRODUCTION

Lowering serum lipid levels is primary to treating and preventing clinically significant cardiovascular (CV) disease. Lipid-altering drugs, especially statins, are among the most widely prescribed drugs in the world. Clinical trials over the past 25 years have demonstrated that statins are well tolerated and prevent major CV events (stroke, myocardial infarction) and CV as well as total mortality in high-risk patients. Lipid-altering agents encompass several classes of drugs that include hydroxy-methyl-glutaryl coenzyme A (HMG-CoA) reductase inhibitors or statins, fibric acid derivatives, bile acid sequestrants, cholesterol absorption inhibitors, nicotinic acid, and proprotein convertase subtilisin/kexin type 9 (PCSK9) inhibitors. These drugs differ with respect to mechanism of action and to the degree and type of lipid-lowering. In addition to lipid-lowering properties, these drugs have additional pleiotropic effects. The pleiotropic benefits may be mediated by a reduction in systemic inflammation, endothelial dysfunction and platelet hyper-reactivity. Some of the noncardiovascular effects are beneficial, whereas others may be harmful.

Many primary care physicians face the challenge of identifying a therapeutic regimen that not only achieves desired lipid goals, but also is well tolerated by the patient. This chapter aims to provide a balanced evaluation and critique of the available evidence on endocrine effects of lipid-lowering drugs.

ENDOCRINE EFFECTS OF LIPID-LOWERING DRUGS

Lipid-lowering Drugs and Diabetes

Statins have effects on glucose metabolism that might influence the development of diabetes mellitus in nondiabetics or affect glycemic control in patients with existing diabetes. Statin therapy confers a small increased risk of new-onset diabetes mellitus (NODM) and the risk is greater with more intensive statin regimens. In 2012, the US Food and Drug Administration added a statement to the label of statins indicating that increase in glycated hemoglobin (HbA1c) and fasting glucose levels have been reported with statin use.[1]

Clinical trials and meta-analyses have clearly shown that statins can increase the incidence of NODM. A meta-analysis of five randomized controlled trials (RCTs) (n = 32,752), done in 2011 found an increased risk of incident diabetes with intensive statin therapy compared with moderate statin therapy (OR 1.12, CI 1.04–1.22) with little or no heterogeneity across trials. This translates into approximately one additional case of diabetes for every 500 patients treated with intensive rather than moderate statin therapy.[2] A 2015 meta-analysis confirmed these results both for the risk of diabetes with statins versus placebo (OR 1.11, CI 1.03–1.20) and for intensive versus moderate-intensity statin therapy (OR 1.12, CI 1.04–1.22). This study also included a Mendelian randomization study that found that decreased genetic HMG-CoA reductase activity is associated with a higher risk of type 2 diabetes (T2D).[3]

In a retrospective cohort study using electronic health records from South East Asia, 8,265 statin-exposed patients were compared with 33,060 matched nonexposed individuals.[4] The comparative risks for NODM with various statins (atorvastatin, fluvastatin, pitavastatin, pravastatin, rosuvastatin, and simvastatin) were estimated by both statin exposure versus matched nonexposed and within-class comparisons. The incidence of NODM among statin-exposed group [6.000 per 1000 patient-years (PY)] was higher than that of nonexposed group (3.244 per 1000 PY). The hazard ratio of NODM after statin exposure was 1.872 (95% CI, 1.432–2.445). When comparing hazard ratios between statins, pitavastatin and pravastatin were associated with a lower risk for NODM. Additionally, in another meta-analysis, pitavastatin had no adverse effect on glucose metabolism or glycemic status.[5]

The increased diabetes mellitus risk seen with statins and other lipid-lowering therapies is dose-dependent and mainly observed in patients with underlying abnormalities of carbohydrate homeostasis such as prediabetes or those at greater risk due to abdominal obesity, metabolic syndrome or a family history of diabetes.

The effect of PCSK9 inhibitors on glucose metabolism seems to be less evident and while studies have demonstrated a slight increase in fasting glucose and HbA1c, these agents have not been associated with increased risk of NODM.[6] Other lipid-lowering drugs also have variable effect on glycemia with niacin demonstrating both an increased risk of NODM as well as a potential to worsen glycemic control in diabetics.[7] Ezetimibe, fibrates or bile acid sequestrants seem to have a small but insignificant effect on glycemia.[7] On the other hand, colesevelam has been demonstrated to improve insulin sensitivity and has modest effect in improving glycemic control.[8]

What are the Proposed Mechanisms for Diabetes with Statin Use?

All lipid-lowering drugs associated with a detrimental effect on carbohydrate homeostasis (statins, ezetimibe, and PCSK9 inhibitors) share a common mechanism of hypolipidemic effect. They act via increasing the expression of low-density lipoprotein receptors (LDLRs), including an up-regulation of LDLRs in the pancreatic β-cells. This further leads to lipid accumulation within the β-cell and β-cell dysfunction. The above hypothesis is supported by a study reporting the prevalence of T2D in patients with familial hypercholesterolemia (FH), who have decreased LDLR expression.[9] The prevalence of T2D in patients with FH is lower compared with their unaffected relatives. However, low LDL levels in familial hypobetalipoproteinemia were not associated with risk of diabetes.[10] Therefore, enhanced LDL clearance cannot clearly explain the diabetogenic potential of statins.

Hence, other mechanisms affecting insulin resistance, insulin secretion, or both likely explain statin-induced dysglycemia. Statins may interfere with insulin signaling in several ways:[11]
- Affect insulin secretion directly or indirectly by their effect on calcium channels in pancreatic β-cells
- Reduce glucose transporter type 4 translocation
- Decrease important downstream products like coenzyme Q (CoQ), farnesyl pyrophosphate (FPP), geranylgeranyl pyrophosphate (GGPP)–depletion results in impaired insulin signaling.

These are summarized in figure 1. The underlying mechanism for dysglycemia is not completely understood and even within the class of statins, there are differences in the diabetogenic potential. Pravastatin and pitavastatin exhibit a neutral or even a beneficial effect on glucose homeostasis.[12] It is interesting to note that lipid-lowering drugs that decrease LDL-cholesterol (LDL-C) without directly interfering with LDLR expression, such as cholesteryl ester transfer protein inhibitors, did not have detrimental effect on carbohydrate homeostasis.[13]

The bile acid sequestrant, colesevelam, activates farnesoid X receptor (bile acid receptor), that reduces the expression of gluconeogenic enzymes such as glucose-6-phosphatase and phosphoenolpyruvate carboxykinase. Colesevelam has been shown to result in modest improvements in insulin sensitivity and glycemic control.[14]

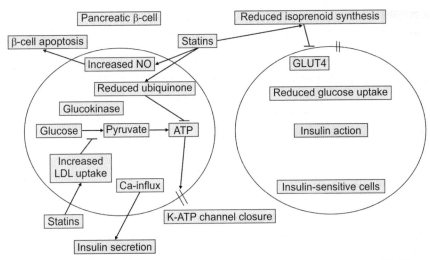

ATP, adenosine triphosphate; GLUT4, glucose transporter type 4; NO, nitric oxide; Ca, calcium; K-ATP, ATP sensitive potassium channel; HMG-CoA, 3-hydroxy-3-methylglutaryl coenzyme A; LDL, low density lipoprotein.

FIG. 1: Mechanism of diabetogenic effects of statins. Statins act by upregulation of LDL receptors on cell surface and increase the uptake of LDL in pancreatic β-cells. The increased intracellular lipid content inhibits glucokinase and ATP generation. Statins inhibit HMG-CoA reductase and reduce the availability of downstream ubiquinone, which further leads to reduced intracellular ATP production. Thereby, they reduce intracellular calcium influx and insulin secretion from the β-cells. An increase in NO production may promote β-cell apoptosis. A reduction in isoprenoid synthesis has been associated with downregulation of GLUT4 transport proteins in insulin-sensitive cells such as adipocytes, with a resultant decrease in peripheral glucose uptake and impaired insulin sensitivity seen with the use of statins.

Despite the potential of statins to cause dysglycemia, the CV benefits outweigh their small diabetogenic risk.[15] This risk is seen more in individuals at risk of diabetes and occurs more with higher intensity statin therapy. Therefore, most guidelines still consider statins as the primary therapy for CV risk reduction in diabetic as well as nondiabetic individuals.

Lipid-lowering Drugs and Myopathy

Muscle syndromes associated with statins include myalgias, myopathy, myositis, and muscle injury. The 2014 National Lipid Association Statin Muscle Safety Task Force[16] defines muscle syndromes associated with lipid-lowering drugs as enlisted in table 1.

How Prevalent is Muscle Involvement with Lipid-lowering Drugs?

Information about muscle injury and statins has come from both large clinical trials and observational studies. In a meta-analysis of 26 RCTs, an excess risk of 4 per 10,000 patients treated was found with high intensity statins compared to lower intensity statins.[17] The risk of rhabdomyolysis was 1 per 10,000 people treated with statins. The overall incidence of excess cases of myositis and rhabdomyolysis is estimated at 0.5 and 0.1 per 1000 PY, respectively.[17] No significant risk of rhabdomyolysis was seen in another meta-analysis of 16 trials (68,110 patients) while the relative risk of myalgias without increase in creatine kinase (CK) was 0.99 (0.96–1.03) in 21 studies.[18]

TABLE 1	National Lipid Association Statin Muscle Safety Task Force definition of muscle syndromes with lipid-lowering drugs
Myalgia	A symptom of muscle discomfort, including muscle aches, soreness, stiffness, tenderness, or cramps with or soon after exercise, with a normal creatine kinase (CK) level
Myopathy	Muscle weakness (not due to pain), with or without an elevation in CK level
Myositis	Muscle inflammation
Myonecrosis	Elevation in muscle enzymes compared with either baseline CK levels (while not on statin therapy) or the upper limit of normal that has been adjusted for age, race, and sex • Mild: 3–10-fold elevation in CK • Moderate: 10–50-fold elevation in CK • Severe: 50-fold or greater elevation in CK
Clinical rhabdomyolysis	Myonecrosis with myoglobinuria or acute renal failure (an increase in serum creatinine of least 0.5 mg/dL)

While the rates of significant myopathy and rhabdomyolysis may be low, the overall incidence of muscle complaints in clinical practice and observational studies associated with statins can be high and varies widely, from 0.3 to 33%[19] and this has led to obvious concerns.[19] In a cross-sectional observational study of 3,580 adults in the US National Health and Nutrition Examination Survey,[20] the prevalence of any musculoskeletal pain in the previous 30 days in statin users and nonusers was 22.0% and 16.7%, respectively (OR 1.50, 18.0 to 26.7%; p = 0.01).

What is the Time Course of Muscle Events?

The onset of muscle symptoms is usually within weeks to months after the initiation of statin therapy but may occur at any time during treatment. Myalgias and weakness resolve, and serum CK concentrations return to normal over days to weeks after discontinuation of the drug.

What are the Risk Factors for Myopathy?

The risks related to myopathy are associated with following factors:[21]
- Statin characteristics: The ability to cause muscle injury appears to differ among statins. The more hydrophilic statins, pravastatin and rosuvastatin, may have less penetration into muscle than the more lipophilic statins. In addition, pravastatin, fluvastatin, and pitavastatin are also less likely to be involved with drug interactions as they are not metabolized by cytochrome P450 3A4 (CYP3A4)
- Co-existing disorders: Statin-associated myopathy is more common in patients with co-existing hypothyroidism, acute or chronic renal failure, obstructive liver disease and amyotrophic lateral sclerosis (ALS) or conditions that mimic ALS
- Vigorous exercise: Vigorous unaccustomed exercise in those on statins may increase the risk for muscle injury. Patients who are taking statins need not eliminate exercise. This risk can be mitigated by graduated exercise training program.

TABLE 2 Drugs increasing the risk of statin-associated myopathy

Drugs	Mechanism of effect
Cyclosporine, macrolide antibiotics (erythromycin), systemic-azole, antifungals, HIV/HCV protease inhibitors (including ritonavir)	Drugs and substances that inhibit cytochrome P450 3A4 (CYP3A4) can increase the risk of statin myopathy due to lovastatin, simvastatin, and to a lesser extent atorvastatin[18]
Calcium channel blockers (CCB)	Non-dihydropyridine CCBs, diltiazem and verapamil, are moderate inhibitors of CYP3A4 metabolism. Simvastatin at a dose of 20–80 mg/day causes a 0.6% incidence of myopathy in patients also treated with verapamil. Amlodipine does not inhibit CYP3A4 but is a competitive CYP3A4 substrate. Increased concentrations of simvastatin are observed when taken with amlodipine
Fibrates	Independent association with muscle toxicity. Combination of lovastatin and atorvastatin with gemfibrozil increases the risk of muscle toxicity, as high as 1–5%
Colchicine	Infrequent adverse effect, particularly in the setting of renal insufficiency

HIV, human immunodeficiency virus; HCV, hepatitis C virus.

- Vitamin D deficiency: Few small studies have suggested that low vitamin D levels may be associated with statin myopathy.[22] Symptomatic improvements have been reported with vitamin D supplementation, but there is no evidence from RCTs. At present the evidence is insufficient to support testing for vitamin D deficiency in patients with statin-induced myalgia. However, in the patient known to be vitamin D deficient with a history of statin intolerance, re-challenging with a statin once vitamin D levels are replete is a reasonable strategy
- Concurrent drug therapy: There are increased chances of myopathy in patients receiving concurrent drugs, particularly those that inhibit CYP3A4 as well as with fibrates. These are enlisted in table 2. It is important to understand that there exist differences in the metabolism of various statins. Simvastatin, lovastatin and to a lesser extent, atorvastatin, are metabolized by CYP3A4. Fluvastatin is partly dependent upon cytochrome P450 2C9 metabolism while rosuvastatin, pitavastatin and pravastatin are cleared primarily by non-CYP-450 transformations.

Fibrates have also been associated with significant muscle toxicity and more pronounced effects on those already taking statins. Gemfibrozil should not be started concurrently in patients taking a statin. It causes a high risk of rhabdomyolysis. Myopathy has been rarely reported with ezetimibe monotherapy; however, risk may be increased with concomitant use of statin or fibrates.

Does the Switching of Statins Help in Myopathy?

Pravastatin, fluvastatin, and pitavastatin appear to have much less intrinsic muscle toxicity than other statins. It is advised to switch the patient to one of the above statins once symptoms have resolved off statin therapy.[23]

What is the Role of Alternate-day Dosing of Statins?

Alternate-day dosing may improve the tolerability of statins in patients experiencing myalgia, and this strategy appears to have equal LDL-C lowering efficacy. It can be useful in patients not tolerating daily statin therapy.[24]

Lipid-lowering Drugs and Bone Metabolism

In addition to cholesterol lowering and the primary and secondary prevention of cardiovascular disease, statin therapy may be associated with other benefits. Statins have demonstrated osteogenic effects in animals and human osteosarcoma cell lines.[25] Statins promote bone formation and increase bone mineral density, while bone resorption is reduced. Hence, they may increase bone volume, and density, and have the potential to reduce the risk of osteoporotic fractures, particularly in older patients.

Mechanism of Bone Anabolic Effects of Statins

Statins may improve bone health by several mechanisms as depicted in figure 2:
- Promote osteoblast differentiation and osteogenesis
- Inhibit osteoblast apoptosis
- Inhibit osteoclastogenesis.

Statins reduce the synthesis of FPP and GGPP, and this results in increased osteoblast differentiation and osteogenesis. Increase in RAS and its downstream signaling molecules protein kinase B (Akt) and extracellular signal regulated kinase (ERK) results in increased expression of bone morphometric protein 2 (BMP-2), that further promotes osteoblast differentiation. Osteoblast apoptosis is inhibited via transforming growth factor β (TGFβ) and Smad3 pathways. Statins also upregulate the expression of estrogen receptor (ER) and down regulate signaling via receptor activator of nuclear factor κ-B ligand (RANKL)/receptor activator of nuclear factor κ-B (RANK), resulting in reduced osteoclast activity. The net result is an increase in bone formation and reduced bone resorption.[25]

Clinical Evidence of Bone Effects

Clinical studies pertaining to the effect of statins on bone health have yielded conflicting results. Several observational studies suggested that statins have a positive effect on bone health but results from randomized trials have not demonstrated the same.

In some studies, statin therapy was associated with a decrease in fractures or an increase in bone mineral density (BMD).[26] In other studies, there was no decrease in fractures.[27] The Women's Health Initiative study, the largest observational study to address this issue, reported no reduction in fracture rates in postmenopausal statin users compared with nonusers after 4 years of follow-up.[28] In another trial, 82 postmenopausal women were randomly assigned to simvastatin (40 mg/day) or placebo for 1 year. There were no effects of simvastatin on biochemical bone markers or on BMD at the hip or spine; although, an increase in bone density was seen in the forearm.[29] In a meta-analysis of seven trials, statin therapy was found to significantly increase BMD but did not have any effect on fracture risk.[30]

CHAPTER 15: Endocrine Effects of Lipid-lowering Drugs

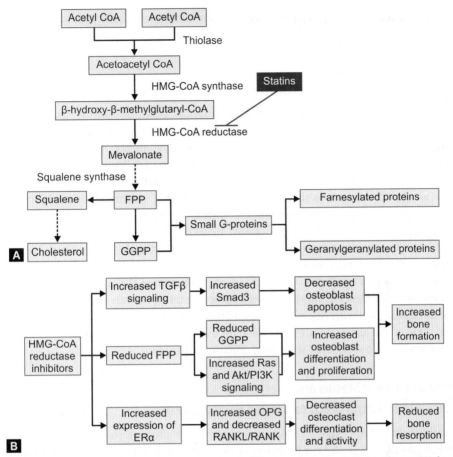

BMP-2, bone morphometric protein 2; ER, estrogen receptor; ERK, extra-cellular signal regulated kinase; FPP, farnesyl pyrophosphate; GGPP, geranyl geranyl pyrophosphate; HMG-CoA, 3-hydroxy-3-methylglutaryl coenzyme A; MAPK, mitogen activated protein kinase; OPG, osteoprotegerin; RANK, receptor activator of nuclear factor κ-B; RANKL, receptor activator of nuclear factor κ-B ligand; TGFβ, transforming growth factor β; Akt, protein kinase B.

FIG. 2: Proposed mechanisms of bone anabolic effects of HMG-CoA reductase inhibitors. **A,** Reduced generation of FPP and GGPP: Statins inhibit HMG-CoA reductase, the rate limiting step in cholesterol biosynthesis and reduce the synthesis of mevalonate with a resultant decrease in FPP generation. While FPP is converted to cholesterol by the action of squalene synthase, FPP also acts as an intermediatory for other downstream effects; FPP is a component of fanesylated proteins formed from small G-proteins and in addition, leads to formation of GGPP and geranylated proteins; **B,** Increased osteogenesis and reduced osteoclast activity: Statins block the generation of mevalonate by inhibiting HMG-CoA reductase. This results in reduced synthesis of FPP and GGPP. Both FPP and GGPP negatively regulate osteogenesis and statins may stimulate osteogenesis by reducing their production. FPP and GGPP activate small G-proteins including Ras/Rap, Rho/Rap, Rab, Ran, and Arf that regulate several cellular processes including cytoskeletal formation and osteogenesis. While statins inhibit Rho, they activate Ras and its downstream signaling molecules Akt and ERK. This results in increased expression of BMP-2 and MAPK that stimulate differentiation of mesenchymal stem cells into osteoblasts. In addition, they also inhibit osteoblast apoptosis by increasing the expression of Smad3 protein downstream of TGFβ signaling pathway, independent of BMP signaling. Statins inhibit osteoclast activity by increasing the expression of ERα in the bone. Additionally, they also regulate the OPG/RANKL/RANK pathway that plays a key role in osteoclastogenesis; RANK guides the differentiation and proliferation of osteoclasts and increases bone resorption while simultaneously reducing bone formation. Statins have been shown to reduce RANKL signaling, thus reducing bone resorption. The net result is an increase in bone formation and reduced bone resorption.

One reason why statins have failed to demonstrate clinically meaningful bone anabolic effects is that currently available statins target liver and do not reach significant concentration in the bone.

Lipid-lowering Drugs and Erectile Dysfunction

Several studies have investigated the association between statins and erectile dysfunction, with the hypothesis that statins improve erectile function through beneficial effects on the endothelium and increased availability of nitric oxide.[31] The Erectile Dysfunction and Statins Trial randomly assigned 173 patients with erectile dysfunction to simvastatin 40 mg or placebo and followed participants for a median of 30 weeks. Treatment with simvastatin produced a statistically nonsignificant improvement on an erectile dysfunction index.[32] Two recent RCTs in men with erectile dysfunction initially unresponsive to sildenafil suggested that atorvastatin could improve erectile responsiveness to sildenafil.[33,34] On the other hand, there is the concern that statins could theoretically worsen erectile function in some men through decreased synthesis of testosterone.[35] However, the same has not been demonstrated in a recent meta-analysis, involving 24,661 statin users where statins were not associated with risk of new-onset erectile dysfunction.[36]

In view of the above, at present based on available data, no definitive conclusion can be drawn on the effect of statins on erectile dysfunction.

Potential Effect of Statins and Other Lipid-lowering Drugs on Steroid Hormogenesis

Lipid-lowering drugs have a theoretical potential to affect steroid hormogenesis in adrenal glands and gonads as they reduce serum cholesterol, which is a precursor of the steroid biosynthetic pathway. Statins reduce androgen production from theca-interstitial cells of the ovaries and hence, they have demonstrated beneficial effects on androgen levels and luteinizing hormone (LH)/follicle-stimulating hormone (FSH) ratio in women with PCOS.[37] While this has been associated with clinical improvement in some studies, most studies have failed to demonstrate benefits on hyperandrogenism or ovulation and statins are not recommended for routine use in PCOS women.

In males, some studies reported reduction in LH secretion and testosterone production.[38] Concern has been raised about a possible deleterious effect of statins on male fertility, but studies have not reported any negative effect on gonadal or sexual health in men or women so far.[39,40] However, it is prudent to assess the long-term effects of statins on gonadal and sexual functions.

On the contrary, a systematic review of seven studies found a significant increase in serum cortisol concentrations following statin treatment with lipophilic (atorvastatin, simvastatin, lovastatin) but not hydrophilic statins.[41] The clinical significance of this effect is not known. While statins may reduce postganglionic sympathetic nervous activity in hypertensive subjects, no effect on plasma epinephrine levels has been demonstrated.[42]

Other Endocrine Effects

Bile Acid Sequestrants
- Cholestyramine increases fecal excretion of thyroid hormones by reducing their enterohepatic circulation and has been used in hyperthyroidism[43]
- Chronic use of bile acid sequestrants may lead to development of hyperchloremic acidosis especially with cholestyramine and colestipol.

Niacin
- Can lead to troublesome flushing
- Induces hyperuricemia and may precipitate acute gouty arthritis.

Fenofibrate
It may have a potential beneficial role in management of diabetic neuropathy and retinopathy independent of its lipid-lowering effect.[44]

Clofibrate
It can cause syndrome of inappropriate antidiuretic hormone secretion and has been used in management of nephrogenic diabetes insipidus.[45]

Thyromimetics
Eprotirome is a thyroid hormone analog that has minimal uptake in nonhepatic tissue. Eprotirome reduces LDL-C in a dose-dependent fashion; at a dose of 100 μg daily, LDL-C was reduced by 32%, compared with a 7% reduction with placebo. Similar changes were seen in levels of triglycerides, lipoprotein (a), and apolipoprotein B. Eprotirome did not appear to produce clinical hyperthyroidism, hypothyroidism, or had adverse effects on the heart or bone.[46]

CONCLUSION

Lipid-lowering therapy is proven to reduce the risk of CV disease and associated events. Accumulating evidence from basic research and clinical trials indicates that lipid-lowering drugs have a plethora of endocrine effects. The clinical relevance of some of these effects is recognized, and ongoing studies will be able to answer many of the remaining questions in near future.

REFERENCES

1. FDA drug safety communication: Important safety label changes to cholesterol lowering statin drugs. Available from: http://www.fda.gov/Drugs/DrugSafety/ucm293101.htm
2. Preiss D, Seshasai SR, Welsh P, et al. Risk of incident diabetes with intensive-dose compared with moderate-dose statin therapy: A meta-analysis. JAMA. 2011;305(24):2556.
3. Swerdlow DI, Preiss D, Kuchenbaecker KB, et al. HMG-coenzyme A reductase inhibition, type 2 diabetes, and bodyweight: Evidence from genetic analysis and randomised trials. Lancet. 2015;385(9965):351.
4. Yoon D, Sheen SS, Lee S, et al. Statins and risk for new-onset diabetes mellitus: A real-world cohort study using a clinical research database. Medicine. 2016;95(46):e5429.

5. Vallejo-Vaz AJ, Kondapally Seshasai SR, Kurogi K, et al. Effect of pitavastatin on glucose, HbA1c and incident diabetes: A meta-analysis of randomized controlled clinical trials in individuals without diabetes. Atherosclerosis. 2015;241(2):409-18.
6. de Carvalho LSF, Campos AM, Sposito AC. Proprotein convertase subtilisin/kexin type 9 (PCSK9) inhibitors and incident type 2 diabetes: A systematic review and meta-analysis with over 96,000 patient-years. Diabetes Care. 2018;41(2):364-367.
7. Collins PD, Sattar N. Glycaemic effects of non-statin lipid-lowering therapies. Curr Cardiol Rep. 2016;18(12):133.
8. Zafrir B, Jain M. Lipid-lowering therapies, glucose control and incident diabetes: Evidence, mechanisms and clinical implications. Cardiovasc Drugs Ther. 2014;28(4):361-77.
9. Besseling J, Kastelein JJ, Defesche JC, et al. Association between familial hypercholesterolemia and prevalence of type 2diabetes mellitus. JAMA. 2015;313(10):1029-36.
10. Noto D, Arca M, Tarugi P, et al. Association between familial hypobetalipoproteinemia and the risk of diabetes. Is this the other side of the cholesterol-diabetes connection? A systematic review of literature. Acta Diabetol. 2017;54(2):111-22.
11. Brault M, Ray J, Gomez YH, et al. Statin treatment and new-onset diabetes: A review of proposed mechanisms. Metabolism. 2014;63(6):735-45.
12. Laakso M, Kuusisto J. Diabetes secondary to treatment with statins. Curr Diab Rep. 2017;17(2):10.
13. Filippatos TD, Klouras E, Barkas F, et al. Cholesteryl ester transfer protein inhibitors: Challenges and perspectives. Expert Rev Cardiovasc Ther. 2016;14(8):953-96.
14. Fonseca VA, Handelsman Y, Staels B. Colesevelam lowers glucose and lipid levels in type 2 diabetes: The clinical evidence. Diabetes Obes Metab. 2010;12(5):384-92.
15. Agarwala A, Kulkarni S, Maddox T. The association of statin therapy with incident diabetes: Evidence, mechanisms, and recommendations. Curr Cardiol Rep. 2018;20(7):50.
16. Rosenson RS, Baker SK, Jacobson TA, et al. An assessment by the Statin Muscle Safety Task Force: 2014 update. J Clin Lipidol. 2014;8(3 Suppl):S58-71.
17. Baigent C, Blackwell L, Emberson J, et al. Efficacy and safety of more intensive lowering of LDL cholesterol: A meta-analysis of data from 170 000 participants in 26 randomised trials. Lancet. 2010;376:1670-81.
18. Kashani A, Phillips CO, Foody JM, et al. Risks associated with statin therapy: A systematic overview of randomized clinical trials. Circulation. 2006;114:2788-97.
19. McKenney JM, Davidson MH, Jacobson TA. Final conclusions and recommendations of the National Lipid Association Statin Safety Assessment Task Force. Am J Cardiol. 2006;97(8A):89C-94C.
20. Buettner C, Davis RB, Leveille SG, et al. Prevalence of musculoskeletal pain and statin use. J Gen Intern Med. 2008;23:1182-6.
21. Chatzizisis YS, Koskinas KC, Misirli G, et al. Risk factors and drug interactions predisposing to statin-induced myopathy: Implications for risk assessment, prevention and treatment. Drug Saf. 2010;33(3):171.
22. Gupta A, Thompson PD. The relationship of vitamin D deficiency to statin myopathy. Atherosclerosis. 2011;215(1):23.
23. Joy TR, Hegele RA. Narrative review: Statin-related myopathy. Ann Intern Med. 2009;150(12):858.
24. Awad K, Mikhailidis DP, Toth PP, et al. Efficacy and safety of alternate-day versus daily dosing of statins: A systematic review and meta-analysis. Cardiovasc Drugs Ther. 2017;31(4):419.
25. Ruan F, Zheng Q, Wang J. Mechanisms of bone anabolism regulated by statins. Biosci Rep. 2012;32(6):511-9.
26. Wang PS, Solomon DH, Mogun H, et al. HMG-CoA reductase inhibitors and the risk of hip fractures in elderly patients. JAMA. 2000;283(24):3211.
27. El-Sohemy A. Statin drugs and the risk of fracture. JAMA. 2000;284(15):1921.
28. LaCroix AZ, Cauley JA, Pettinger M, et al. Statin use, clinical fracture, and bone density in postmenopausal women: Results from the Women's Health Initiative Observational Study. Ann Intern Med. 2003;139(2):97.
29. Rejnmark L, Buus NH, Vestergaard P, et al. Effects of simvastatin on bone turnover and BMD: A 1-year randomized controlled trial in postmenopausal osteopenic women. J Bone Miner Res. 2004;19(5):737.

30. Wang Z, Li Y, Zhou F, et al. Effects of statins on bone mineral density and fracture risk: A PRISMA-compliant systematic review and meta-analysis. Medicine (Baltimore). 2016;95(22):e3042.
31. La Vignera S, Condorelli RA, Vicari E, et al. Statins and erectile dysfunction: A critical summary of current evidence. J Androl. 2012;33:552-8.
32. Trivedi D, Kirby M, Wellsted DM, et al. Can simvastatin improve erectile function and health-related quality of life in men aged ≥40 years with erectile dysfunction? Results of the Erectile Dysfunction and Statins Trial. BJU Int. 2013;111(2):324.
33. El-Sisi AA, Hegazy SK, Salem KA, et al. Atorvastatin improves erectile dysfunction in patients initially irresponsive to sildenafil by the activation of endothelial nitric oxide synthase. Int J Impot Res. 2013;25(4):143.
34. Dadkhah F, Safarinejad MR, Asgari MA, et al. Atorvastatin improves the response to sildenafil in hypercholesterolemic men with erectile dysfunction not initially responsive to sildenafil. Int J Impot Res. 2010;22(1):51-60.
35. Corona G, Boddi V, Balercia G, et al. The effect of statin therapy on testosterone levels in subjects consulting for erectile dysfunction. J Sex Med. 2010;7:1547-56.
36. Elgendy AY, Elgendy IY, Mahmoud AN, et al. Statin use in men and new onset of erectile dysfunction: A systematic review and meta-analysis. Am J Med. 2018;131(4):387-394.
37. Cassidy-Vu L, Joe E, Kirk JK. Role of statin drugs for polycystic ovary syndrome. J Family Reprod Health. 2016;10(4):165-75.
38. Feingold K, Brinton EA, Grunfeld C. The effect of endocrine disorders on lipids and lipoproteins. In: De Groot LJ, Choruses G, Dungan K, et al., editors. Endotext [Internet]. South Dartmouth (MA): MDText.com, Inc.; 2000-2017 Feb 24.
39. Baspınar O, Bayram F, Korkmaz S, et al. The effects of statin treatment on adrenal and sexual function and nitric oxide levels in hypercholesterolemic male patients treated with a statin. J Clin Lipidol. 2016;10(6):1452-61.
40. Ali SK, Reveles KR, Davis R, et al. The association of statin use and gonado-sexual function in women: A retrospective cohort analysis. J Sex Med. 2015;12(1):83-92.
41. Sahebkar A, Rathouska J, Simental-Mendía LE, et al. Statin therapy and plasma cortisol concentrations: A systematic review and meta-analysis of randomized placebo-controlled trials. Pharmacol Res. 2016;103:17-25.
42. Gomes ME, Tack CJ, Verheugt FW, et al. Sympathoinhibition by atorvastatin in hypertensive patients. Circ J. 2010;74(12):2622-6.
43. Er C, Sule AA. Cholestyramine as monotherapy for Graves' hyperthyroidism. Singapore Med J. 2016; 57(11):644.
44. Sharma N, Ooi JL, Ong J, et al. The use of fenofibrate in the management of patients with diabetic retinopathy: An evidence-based review. Australian Family Physician. 2015; 44(6):367.
45. Kalra S, Zargar AH, Jain SM, et al. Diabetes insipidus: The other diabetes. Indian J Endocrinol Metab. 2016;20(1):9-21.
46. Ladenson PW, Kristensen JD, Ridgway EC, et al. Use of the thyroid hormone analogue eprotirome in statin-treated dyslipidemia. N Engl J Med. 2010;362(10):906.

CHAPTER 16

PCSK-9 Inhibitors: Endocrine Considerations

Sunil K Mishra, Sanjay Kalra, Gagan Priya

ABSTRACT

Lipid-lowering therapies targeting low-density lipoprotein cholesterol (LDL-C) are the mainstay for the management and prevention of atherosclerotic cardiovascular disease (ASCVD). While statins remain the first choice drugs, they are limited in efficacy as well as tolerability. Proprotein convertase subtilisin/kexin type-9 (PCSK-9) inhibitors constitute a new class of very potent lipid-lowering drugs. These drugs have offered new hope of treatment for patients who have genetic hyperlipidemia or are at very high-risk for cardiovascular disease and are not able to reduce their LDL-C level with existing therapies. Recent clinical trials and postmarketing data have provided more information on how these drugs should be used in the treatment of dyslipidemia and the prevention of cardiovascular disease. The available safety profile of these drugs gives enough confidence to clinicians for its use in high risk ASCVD patients. The cost of available PCSK-9 inhibitors is one major limiting factor for many eligible patients. However, more research is needed to understand the inter-relationship between various hormones and PCSK-9 and the effect of PCSK-9 inhibitors beyond lipid-lowering.

INTRODUCTION

Lipid-lowering therapies targeting low-density lipoprotein cholesterol (LDL-C) are the mainstay for the management and prevention of atherosclerotic cardiovascular disease (ASCVD). Since the publication of the Scandinavian Simvastatin Survival Study, statins or inhibitors of 3-hydroxy-3-methyl-glutaryl-coenzyme A reductase have become standard of care for addressing ASCVD. For each 38.6 mg/dL (1 mmol/L) reduction in LDL-C, ASCVD risk is reduced by 21%.[1] Therefore, moderate to high intensity statins are recommended.

However, statin use is limited by its adverse effects, mainly myalgias, myositis, and hepatotoxicity. It is now well recognized that cardiovascular disease (CVD) events continue to occur despite ongoing statin therapy. The LDL-C lowering potential of statins is particularly limited in individuals with familial hypercholesterolemia (FH), who harbor a very high cardiovascular risk. Further, up-titration of statin therapy does not result in linear lowering in LDL-C. Therefore, some patients may require addition of other drugs that reduce LDL-C, such as ezetimibe or PCSK-9 inhibitors. These drugs have been found to lower ASCVD events in high-risk populations.

Proprotein convertase subtilisin/kexin type-9 (PCSK-9) inhibitors constitute a new class of very potent lipid-lowering drugs. Most lipid-lowering drugs can have significant effects on the endocrine system, some of which are desirable such as improvement in bone health with statins and improvement in glycemic control with colsevelam and saroglitazar, while others can be detrimental, such as the risk of myopathy and diabetes with statins.[2] Since PCSK-9 inhibitors are relatively newer drugs, it is important to understand their interaction with the endocrine physiology. In this chapter, we focus on the endocrine effects of this novel class of drugs.

PCSK-9 INHIBITORS: MECHANISM OF ACTION

The PCSK-9 belongs to the family of proprotein convertases, which are serine convertases involved in the cleavage and activation of several protein substrates including precursor proteins, growth factors, hormones, receptors, and transmembrane proteins.[3] It is encoded by the *PCSK-9* gene on chromosome 1 and is primarily expressed in and secreted from the liver. It is involved in the regulation of the LDL receptor (LDLR) expression.

The LDLR binds to the LDL particles and the LDL-LDLR complex is then internalized from the extracellular fluid into the hepatocyte or other cells within an endosome. Inside the endosome, there occurs a conformational change in the LDLR causing it to release LDL, which then undergoes degradation. The LDLR is recycled back to the cell membrane for binding to new LDL particles. The PCSK-9 is released by hepatocytes, rapidly undergoes intra-endoplasmic reticulum auto-catalysis and becomes an active protein. This active form of PCSK-9 now binds to the LDLR, and induces its lysosomal degradation, thereby reducing the expression of LDLR on hepatocyte cell membrane. By this mechanism, PCSK-9 reduces the clearance of plasma LDL-C.[3] It has been demonstrated that PCSK-9 gain-of-function mutations result in high LDL-C, increased ASCVD and FH.[4]

In the absence of PCSK-9, there is reduced degradation of LDLR and greater numbers of LDLR are transported to plasma membrane to bind to LDL-C and increase its clearance.[5] In fact, the loss-of-function mutations in PCSK-9 were associated with low LDL-C and fewer ASCVD events.[4] This paved the way for development of inhibitors of PCSK-9 activity, with a potential for significant lowering of LDL-C and ASCVD risk. The mechanism of action of PCSK-9 inhibitors is depicted in figure 1.

The effect of PCSK-9 however is not mediated via LDLR alone. The degradation of VLDL receptor, apolipoprotein E (apoE) receptor 2, CD36 and possibly LRP1 (low density lipoprotein receptor-related protein 1) is also increased by PCSK-9; CD36 is involved in the absorption of free fatty acids in intestinal cells and adipocytes. The PCSK9 also affects degradation of NPC1L1 (Niemann-Pick C1-like protein 1) involved in cholesterol absorption.[5] Other organs where PCSK-9 is expressed include small intestine, adrenals, pancreas, central nervous system, and kidneys.

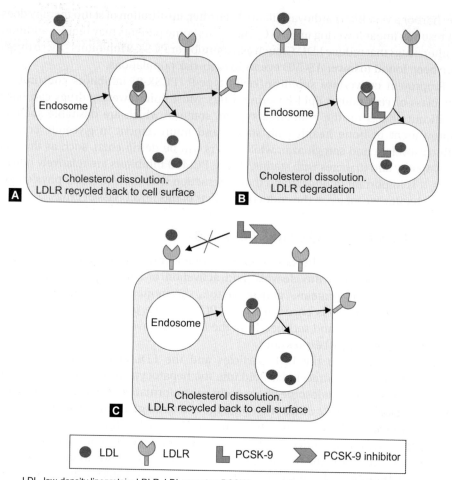

LDL, low-density lipoprotein; LDLR, LDL receptor; PCSK9, proprotein convertase subtilisin/ kexin type 9.

FIG. 1: Mechanism of Action of PCSK-9 Inhibitors. **A,** LDLR binds to the LDL particles and the LDL-LDLR complex is then internalized from the extracellular fluid into the hepatocyte or other cells within an endosome. Inside the endosome, there occurs a conformational change in the LDLR causing it to release LDL, which then undergoes degradation. The LDLR is recycled back to the cell membrane for binding to new LDL particles. PCSK9 is released by hepatocytes, rapidly undergoes intra-endoplasmic reticulum auto-catalysis and becomes an active protein; **B,** PCSK9 undergoes auto-catalysis in the endoplasmic reticulum and the active form of PCSK9 now binds to the LDLR, and induces its lysosomal degradation, thereby reducing the expression of LDLR on hepatocyte cell membrane. By this mechanism, PCSK-9 reduces the clearance of plasma LDL-C; **C,** PCSK9 inhibitors prevent the binding of PCSK9 to the LDLR and prevents its degradation. As a result, greater number of LDLRs are transported to the plasma membrane to bind to LDL-C and increase its clearance. By this mechanism, PCSK9 inhibitors lead to reduced serum cholesterol levels

The synthesis of PCSK-9 is controlled by SREBP-2 (sterol regulatory element binding protein 2), a membrane transcription factor that is involved in cholesterol metabolism. When there is deficiency of intracellular cholesterol, SREBP-2 interacts acts on the promoter of PCSK-9 and LDLR, leading to increased expression of both proteins.[5] Another factor affecting PCSK-9 expression is HNF-1α (hepatocyte nuclear

TABLE 1 PCSK-9 inhibitors in clinical development

Mechanism of PCSK-9 inhibition	Drug class	Agents
Prevent binding of PCSK-9 to LDLR	Monoclonal anti-PCSK-9 antibodies	• Alirocumab • Evolocumab • Bococizumab
	Imitation of EGF-A domain of LDLR – mimetic peptides	Adnectins
Inhibit PCSK-9 mRNA expression	Antisense oligonucleotides	
	Small interfering RNA (siRNA)	Inclisiran
Inhibition of PCSK-9 activity	Inhibitors of PCSK-9 auto-catalytic sites	

EGF-A, epidermal growth factor-like repeat A; LDLR, low-density lipoprotein receptor; PCSK-9, proprotein convertase subtilisin/kexin type-9.

factor 1 homeobox A), but it does not affect LDLR expression directly. Statins act to stimulate the expression of HNF-1α and increase the production of SREBP-2, leading to increased expression of both LDLR and PCSK-9, that limits their LDL-C lowering efficacy.[4] On the other hand, PCSK-9 inhibitors do not seem to cause an increase in SREBP-2 and have a more potent lipid-lowering effect.

DEVELOPMENT OF PCSK-9 INHIBITORS

In 2007, crystal structure of PCSK-9 was discovered and since 2010, human studies with monoclonal antibodies targeting PCSK-9 were started. They act by binding to the LDLR and blocking the effect of PCSK-9, thereby reducing lysosomal degradation of the LDLR. This results in increased cell surface expression of LDLR and increased hepatic clearance of LDL-C. The postprandial clearance of triglycerides is also increased.[6] Therefore, PCSK-9 inhibitors lead to significant reduction in LDL-C, triglycerides, apoB and even lipoprotein a [Lp(a)], whose levels are not affected by statin use.[7]

Several different strategies are under exploration to inhibit the binding of PCSK-9 to LDLR including nonprotein and peptidomimetic agents, antisense oligonucleotides and antibody-based therapies, as enlisted in table 1. Some of the PCSK-9 inhibitors have already been approved for the management of dyslipidemia while others are in development.[5] Most of these are monoclonal antibodies, such as alirocumab, evolocumab, and bococizumab and administered subcutaneously once in 2 weeks.

Alirocumab (FDA Approved)

In phase I and II studies, alirocumab resulted in a greater than 60% decrease in LDL-C. In phase III randomized, double blinded ODYSSEY trials, it reduced LDL-C by more than 50% in poorly controlled hypercholesterolemia and statin intolerant patients. Similarly, in patients with FH, LDL-C levels were reduced by more than 40%. In long-term results of ODYSSEY trials, significant reduction in major cardiovascular events (MACE) including coronary heart disease (CHD) death, nonfatal myocardial infarction (MI), ischemic stroke or unstable angina requiring hospitalization was noticed.[8]

Evolocumab (FDA Approved)

Evolocumab is another approved PCSK-9 inhibitor. The efficacy of evolocumab in phase I and II studies is similar to that reported in trials of alirocumab. FOURIER, the phase III results of evolocumab were recently published. The drug has shown significant reduction in 4-point MACE (CHD death, nonfatal MI, ischemic stroke or unstable angina requiring hospitalization).[8]

In a meta-analysis of 22 randomized controlled trials including 8833 patients, PCSK-9 inhibitors were associated with significant reduction in LDL-C (mean–48.8%; 95% CI –54.1 to –43.4, I^2 = 94%). The reduction in all-cause death was significant even over short study durations (OR = 0.79; 95% CI 0.17–0.69) and there was a trend towards reduction in cardiovascular events (OR 0.79; 95% CI 0.61–1.02).[9] Their effect on increasing high-density lipoprotein cholesterol (HDL-C) and apoA-1 seems to be very small.

INDICATIONS FOR USE OF PCSK-9 INHIBITORS

The PCSK-9 inhibitors have been approved in patients with homozygous or heterozygous FH, individuals with high CV risk with statin intolerance and in those who are unable to achieve LDL-C targets with statin treatment. They are useful especially in individuals who are intolerant to statins or do not attain LDL-C targets after diet modification and maximally tolerated doses of statins.[10] They are currently approved for use in the following conditions:
- Adults with heterozygous FH
- Adults with homozygous FH
- Adults with clinical ASCVD with additional ASCVD risk
- High-risk patients with statin intolerance.

Familial Hypercholesterolemia

Familial hypercholesterolemia is an autosomal dominant genetic disorder of lipid metabolism with prevalence ranging from 1 in 250 to 1 in 300,000 people for heterozygous and homozygous disorder. Heterozygous FH is characterized by LDL-C levels exceeding 190 mg/dL, xanthelasmas, tendon xanthomas, family history of early ASCVD and positive genetic testing. Untreated heterozygous FH presents with early ASCVD (3–4th decades). In homozygous FH, vascular disease starts in early second decade. The treatment of FH was unsatisfactory prior to PCSK-9 inhibitors even with moderate to high-intensity statins. The PCSK-9 inhibitors significantly reduce LDL-C level by as much as 50–60% in FH population.[3] Recent short-term data of PCSK-9 inhibitors use in FH is encouraging, with lower ASCVD rates. Further, long-term data in this high-risk group will help to understand the CV risk reduction potential of this class of drugs.

Statin-intolerant Individuals

The PCSK-9 inhibitors are useful especially in individuals who are intolerant to statins or do not attain LDL-C targets after diet modification and maximally tolerated doses of statins. The statement "maximally tolerated" statin therapy is not alternative to "statin intolerance". Muscle related symptoms are the main reason for discontinuation of statins. The incidence of statin intolerance varies from 1.5-30%. Recent trials comparing PCSK-9 inhibitors (evolocumab and alirocumab) with and without ezetimibe showed significant decline in LDL-C in patients with PCSK-9 inhibitors. In the GAUSS-3 randomized clinical trial there were greater LDL-C reductions with evolocumab compared with ezetimibe, and this provides definitive evidence that they can be safe alternative to statin therapy.[3]

PHARMACOKINETICS AND PHARMACODYNAMICS OF PCSK-9 INHIBITORS

Alirocumab

Maximal serum drug concentrations are reached in 3-7 days, and steady state is reached after 3-4 doses. Median half-life is between 17 and 20 days. Maximal LDL-C reduction is noticed between 3-15 days. The primary mode of elimination of alirocumab is via saturation of targets and proteolysis, depending on drug concentration. No dose adjustment is needed in mild to moderate renal or liver impairment, whereas no data is currently available in severe renal or liver disease patients.

Evolocumab

Time to reach maximal concentration is 3-4 days. The half-life of evolocumab is between 11-17 days. Maximal reduction in LDL-C is noticed within 14 days. No significant alteration in pharmacokinetics is seen in mild-to-moderate renal or liver impairment. There is no available data regarding its use in severe renal or liver disease patients.

SAFETY AND CONTRAINDICATIONS OF PCSK-9 INHIBITORS

These agents appear to be relatively safe and well tolerated with little propensity to cause drug interactions. Side effects may include injection site reactions such as pain and swelling, nasopharyngitis or flu-like reactions and hypersensitivity reactions. The potential for drug-drug interactions is minimal as they do not affect p450 enzymes, transport proteins or QT interval. There was some concern regarding an increased incidence of neurocognitive events, but these have been allayed in larger trials, despite very low LDL-C.[11] Measurement of fat soluble vitamins and steroid hormones was found no different from comparator drugs.

ENDOCRINE EFFECTS OF PCSK-9 INHIBITORS

While PCSK-9 has gained attention primarily due to its role in lipid homeostasis, it has other functions as well. It regulates glucose homeostasis and may play a role in obesity. It also regulates renal sodium reabsorption and has immunomodulatory and neuroprotective effects. Therefore, like other lipid-lowering therapies, PCSK-9 inhibitors have the potential to have other systemic effects including endocrine effects and these have not been completely elucidated. In this section, we discuss what is currently known about the endocrine aspects of PCSK-9 and PCSK-9 inhibitors.

Carbohydrate Metabolism and Diabetes

Diabetes is commonly associated with atherogenic dyslipidemia and significantly increased cardiovascular risk. The PCSK-9 inhibitors hold promise for ASCVD risk reduction in individuals with diabetes and have demonstrated significant LDL-C lowering efficacy and reduction in CV events in the diabetic population. The ODYSSEY DM-INSULIN trial assessed the efficacy and safety of alirocumab as add-on to maximally tolerated statins in type 1 and type 2 diabetics on insulin at high CV risk. Alirocumab use resulted in significant reductions in LDL-C and non-HDL-C, but not triglycerides.[9] While this translates to a potential for additional CV risk reduction, as was evident from the FOURIER trial, diabetics continue to exhibit higher residual CV risk and therapies that reduce triglyceride-rich lipoproteins (TGLs) merit evaluation.

Glucose and lipid metabolisms converge intracellularly to determine cellular energy balance. It is, therefore, important to understand the interface between PCSK-9 and glucose homeostasis.

Effects of PCSK-9 on Glucose Metabolism

The PCSK-9 acts to reduce LDLR and thereby, reduces cholesterol concentration inside the pancreatic β-cells. The accumulation of cholesterol in β-cells impairs insulin secretion. Hence, PCSK-9 has a somewhat positive protective effect on glucose metabolism. Indeed, individuals with FH have high PCSK-9 levels and have a low prevalence of diabetes.[12] By this logic, PCSK-9 inhibitors have the potential to increase diabetes risk. However, genetic studies in individuals with loss-of-function mutations in PCSK-9 have shown mixed results.

PCSK-9 Inhibitors and the Risk of Diabetes

While PCSK-9 inhibitors have demonstrated the potential to reduce CV risk in diabetic individuals, some concerns have been raised about their potential to affect glucose homeostasis. It has been suggested that PCSK-9 inhibitors may increase the risk of hyperglycemia. Mice deficient in the *PCSK-9* gene had lower insulin and higher glucose concentrations in addition to increased LDLR expression. Deposition of cholesterol in the β-cells was associated with islet inflammation and apoptosis.[13,14] In a pooled analysis of phase III trials, alirocumab did not increase the risk of new-onset diabetes over 6–18 months.[15] Similar results were reported from another meta-analysis of trials including both alirocumab and evolocumab.[16] However, there was a significant, albeit small increase in fasting glucose and glycated hemoglobin compared to placebo.

Effect of Insulin on PCSK-9

Insulin has multiple effects on lipid homeostasis. The effects of insulin on PCSK-9 are somewhat controversial. Insulin regulates the LDLR levels by increasing PCSK-9 expression and LDLR degradation. The PCSK-9 seems to be secreted in an insulin-dependent fashion with increased hepatic PCSK-9 expression being regulated by insulin via SREBP-2.[17] In individuals with uncontrolled diabetes mellitus, elevated PCSK-9 levels are found, and this correlated with the level of glycemic control.[18,19] Elevated PCSK-9 concentrations in diabetics have been inconsistently associated with increased cardiovascular risk.[20] Glucagon, on the other hand, has also been shown to reduce PCSK-9 mRNA expression and increase LDLR expression and has hypolipidemic properties.

Effect of Glucose-lowering Drugs on PCSK-9

Glucagon-like peptide 1 (GLP-1) receptor agonist liraglutide has been shown to suppress the expression of PCSK-9 and HNF-1α in HepG2 cells as well as db/db mice.[21] This was associated with improvements in both glucose and lipid concentrations. Not much is known about the effect of peroxisome proliferator-activated receptor-γ (PPAR-γ) on PCSK-9. In HepG2 cells, PPAR-γ ligands induced PCSK-9 mRNA and protein expression. However, despite an increase in PCSK-9, PPAR-γ activation by pioglitazone did not result in decreased LDLR expression and was associated with reduced total and LDL-C.[22] The effects of PPAR-γ agonists on PCSK-9 merit further study as it may explain the differential effects of various thiazolidinediones on LDL-C levels.

Pituitary–Growth Hormone

Growth hormone (GH)-deficient adults have visceral adiposity and increased total and LDL-C. Triglycerides are also elevated while HDL-C may be reduced. Growth hormone replacement may reverse these lipid abnormalities.[23] Acromegaly, on the other hand, is associated with raised triglycerides and low HDL-C and increase in small dense LDL, apoB, and Lp (a). Treatment of acromegaly with normalization of GH and insulin-like growth factor-1 (IGF-1) levels results in lipid improvements.[24] The indications for use of PCSK-9 inhibitors in individuals with abnormalities of the GH axis would remain the same as for general population. Not much is known about the inter-relationship of PCSK-9 with GH, but possibly, endogenous growth hormone levels are unlikely to affect the efficacy or safety of PCSK-9 inhibitors.

Thyroid Hormones

Thyroid hormones significantly impact lipid and lipoprotein metabolism. They increase the expression of LDLR and increase LDL clearance. Triiodothyronine has also been shown to reduce the activity of PCSK-9, which further contributes to the LDL lowering effects of thyroid hormones.[25] Hypothyroidism results in decreased LDL clearance and is classically associated with increased total and LDL-C, hypertriglyceridemia and raised Lp (a).[26] Serum PCSK-9 levels were found to be significantly elevated in individuals with subclinical hypothyroidism, and these correlated with raised LDL-C. The increase in PCSK-9 levels in hypothyroid patients may be due to raised thyroid-stimulating hormone (TSH), as it has been shown that recombinant human TSH (rh-TSH) caused up regulation of PCSK-9 mRNA and protein levels on HepG2 cells, while TSH receptor blocking antibody K1-70 blunted this effect and caused significant reduction in PCSK-9 expression.[27] On the other hand, hyperthyroid individuals have reduced PCSK-9 activity and may manifest hypobetalipoproteinemia.

Levothyroxine treatment results in significant improvements in lipid parameters with reduction in total cholesterol, LDL-C and triglycerides. The Lp (a) levels may also be reduced. The PCSK-9 inhibitors could be useful in individuals with hypothyroidism who continue to have persistent dyslipidemia even after attaining euthyroxinemia.

Gonadal Hormones

Clearance of LDL decreases with increasing age and LDL-C levels increase by almost 30–50%. This is particularly more prominent in women after menopause. Changes in PCSK-9 levels with age may contribute to this increase in LDL-C. The PCSK-9 levels varies with age and between men and women, and the exact mechanism is not well understood, but may be related to the effect of estrogen on PCSK-9. The PCSK-9 levels are higher in men than in women, but decrease with aging in men. On the other hand, they increase with age in women following menopause.[28] This suggests that estrogen may play a role in the regulation of PCSK-9, while testosterone seems to have no effect.[29] Estrogen reduces PCSK-9 levels and an inverse correlation exists between estradiol and PCSK-9 concentrations in women.[29] Increase in endogenous estrogens during *in vitro* fertilization was associated with reduced plasma levels of PCSK-9 and LDL-C. However, a significant change in PCSK-9 was not seen with hormone replacement therapy in postmenopausal women. Hence, more work is required to understand the inter-relationship between sex hormones and lipid metabolism. Testosterone administration did not seem to influence PCSK-9. However, androgen ablative treatment has been associated with variable effects on PCSK-9 concentrations.[28] Currently, there seem to be no effect of PCSK-9 inhibitors on gonadal hormone synthesis.

Adrenal Hormones

Cholesterol is the precursor for adrenal steroid hormone synthesis and is partly derived by the adrenal cortical cells by uptake via LDLR. This leads to the speculation that PCSK-9 inhibitors might affect adrenal steroidogenesis. However, PCSK-9 has a less significant role in lipid metabolism and LDL uptake regulation in adrenals than liver. Annexin A2 (AnxA2) is expressed in extrahepatic tissues such as adrenals and it acts as a functional inhibitor of PCSK-9. It regulates the LDLR degradation in these tissues. In a single case report, a PCSK-9 deficient subject did not demonstrate adrenal insufficiency.[30] Moreover, in DESCARTES study, evolocumab did not show any impact on adrenal or gonadal steroid hormone levels.[31]

CONCLUSION

The PCSK-9 inhibitors are a new class of very potent LDL-C lowering drugs with a potential of significant reduction in ASCVD risk. These drugs have offered new hope of treatment for patients who have genetic hyperlipidemia or are at very high-risk for CVD and are not able to reduce their LDL-C level with existing therapies.

Recent clinical trials and postmarketing data have provided more information on how these drugs should be used in the treatment of dyslipidemia and the prevention of cardiovascular disease. The available safety profile of these drugs gives enough confidence to clinicians for its use in high-risk ASCVD patients. The cost of available PCSK-9 inhibitors is one major limiting factor for many eligible patients. However, more research is needed to understand the inter-relationship between various hormones and PCSK-9 and the effect of PCSK-9 inhibitors beyond lipid-lowering.

REFERENCES

1. Ference BA, Ginsberg HN, Graham I, et al. Low-density lipoproteins cause atherosclerotic cardiovascular disease. 1. Evidence from genetic, epidemiologic, and clinical studies. A consensus statement from the European Atherosclerosis Society Consensus Panel. Eur Heart J. 2017;38(32):2459-72.
2. Kalra S, Priya G. Lipocrinology - the relationship between lipids and endocrine function. Drugs Context. 2018 ;7:212514.
3. Chaudhary R, Garg J, Shah N, et al. PCSK9 inhibitors: A new era of lipid lowering therapy. World J Cardiol. 2017;9(2):76-91.
4. Smith L, Mosley J, Yates J, et al. The new face of hyperlipidemia management: Proprotein convertase subtilisin/kexin inhibitors (PCSK-9) and their emergent role as an alternative to statin therapy. J Pharm Pharm Sci. 2016;19(1):137-46.
5. Klein-Szanto AJ, Bassi DE. Proprotein convertase inhibition: Paralyzing the cell's master switches. Biochem Pharmacol. 2017;140:8-15.
6. Baum SJ, Cannon CP. PCSK9 inhibitor valuation: A science-based review of the two recent models. Clin Cardiol. 2018;41(4):544-50.
7. Wierzbicki AS, Hardman TC, Viljoen A. Inhibition of pro-protein convertase subtilisin kexin 9 (PCSK-9) as a treatment for hyperlipidaemia. Expert Opin Investig Drugs. 2012;21(5):667-76.
8. Rosenson RS, Hegele RA, Fazio S, et al. The evolving future of PCSK9 inhibitors. J Am Coll Cardiol. 2018;72(3):314-329.
9. Squizzato A, Suter MB, Nerone M, et al. PCSK9 inhibitors for treating dyslipidemia in patients at different cardiovascular risk: A systematic review and a meta-analysis. Intern Emerg Med. 2017;12(7):1043-53.
10. Dadu RT, Ballantyne CM. Lipid lowering with PCSK9 inhibitors. Nature Reviews Cardiology. 2014;11(10):563-75.
11. Wiciński M, Żak J, Malinowski B, et al. PCSK9 signaling pathways and their potential importance in clinical practice. EPMA J. 2017;8(4):391-402.
12. Besseling J, Kastelein JJ, Defesche JC. Lower prevalence of type 2 diabetes in patients with familial hypercholesterolaemia. JAMA. 2015;313(10):108.
13. Mbikay M, Sirois F, Mayne J, et al. PCSK9-deficient mice exhibit impaired glucose tolerance and pancreatic islet abnormalities. FEBS Lett. 2009;584:701-6.
14. Filippatos TD, Filippas-Ntekouan S, Pappa E, et al. PCSK9 and carbohydrate metabolism: A double-edged sword. World J Diabetes. 2017;8(7):311-6.
15. Colhoun HM, Ginsberg HN, Robinson JG, et al. No effect of PCSK9 inhibitor alirocumab on the incidence of diabetes in a pooled analysis from 10 ODYSSEY Phase 3 studies. Eur Heart J. 2016;37(39):2981-9.
16. de Carvalho LSF, Campos AM, Sposito AC. Proprotein convertase subtilisin/kexin type 9 (PCSK9) inhibitors and incident type 2 diabetes: A systematic review and meta-analysis with over 96,000 patient-years. Diabetes Care. 2018;41(2):364-7.
17. Miao J, Mathena PV, Haas ME, et al. Role of insulin in the regulation of proprotein convertase subtilisin/kexin type 9. Arterioscler Thromb Vasc Biol. 2015;35(7):1589-96.
18. Levenson AE, Wadwa RP, Shah AS, et al. PCSK9 is increased in youth with type 1 diabetes. Diabetes Care. 2017;40(7):e85-7.

19. Ibarretxe D, Girona J, Plana N, et al. Circulating PCSK9 in patients with type 2 diabetes and related metabolic disorders. Clin Investig Arterioscler. 2016;28(2):71-8.
20. El Khoury P, Roussel R, Fumeron F, et al. Plasma proprotein-convertase-subtilisin/kexin type 9 (PCSK9) and cardiovascular events in type 2 diabetes. Diabetes Obes Metab. 2018;20(4):943-53.
21. Yang SH, Xu RX, Cui CJ, et al. Liraglutide downregulates hepatic LDL receptor and PCSK9 expression in HepG2 cells and db/db mice through a HNF-1α dependent mechanism. Cardiovasc Diabetol. 2018;17(1):48.
22. Duan Y, Chen Y, Hu W, et al. Peroxisome proliferator-activated receptor γ activation by ligands and dephosphorylation induces proprotein convertase subtilisin kexin type 9 and low density lipoprotein receptor expression. J Biol Chem. 2012;287(28):23667-77.
23. Møller N, Gjedsted J, Gormsen L, et al. Effects of growth hormone on lipid metabolism in humans. Growth Hormone & IGF Research. 2003;13:S18-21.
24. Lind S, Rudling M, Ericsson S, et al. Growth hormone induces low-density lipoprotein clearance but not bile acid synthesis in humans. Arterioscler Thromb Vasc Biol. 2004;24:349-56.
25. Bonde Y, Breuer O, Lütjohann D, et al. Thyroid hormone reduces PCSK9 and stimulates bile acid synthesis in humans. J Lipid Res. 20141;55(11):2408-15.
26. Rizos CV, Elisaf MS, Liberopoulos EN. Effects of thyroid dysfunction on lipid profile. Open Cardiovasc Med J. 2011;5:76-84.
27. Gong Y, Ma Y, Ye Z, et al. Thyroid stimulating hormone exhibits the impact on LDLR/LDL-c via up-regulating hepatic PCSK9 expression. Metabolism. 2017;76:32-41.
28. Ooi TC, Raymond A, Cousins M, et al. Relationship between testosterone, estradiol and circulating PCSK9: Cross-sectional and interventional studies in humans. Clin Chim Acta. 2015;446:97-104.
29. Ghosh M, Gälman C, Rudling M, et al. Influence of physiological changes in endogenous estrogen on circulating PCSK9 and LDL cholesterol. J Lipid Res. 2015;56(2):463-9.
30. Cariou B, Benoit I, Le May C. Preserved adrenal function in fully PCSK9-deficient subject. Int J Cardiol. 2014;176(2):499-500.
31. Blom DJ, Djedjos CS, Monsalvo ML, et al. Effects of evolocumab on vitamin E and steroid hormone levels: Results from the 52-week, phase 3, double-blind, randomized, placebo-controlled DESCARTES study. Circ Res. 2015;117(8):731-41.

Index

Page numbers followed by, *b* refer to box, *f* refer to figure, *fc* refer to flowchart, and *t* refer to table.

A

Acanthosis nigricans 110
Acetyl-CoA carboxylase 44
Acromegaly 6, 15, 64, 66, 126
Adenosine
   monophosphate-activated protein kinase 21, 22, 153
   triphosphate 33, 40, 163
Adipocyte 34, 87, 98
   dysfunction 91*f*
Adipocytokines 73
Adipogenesis 22
Adipokines 77, 79*f*
   physiological function 77*t*
Adiponectin 77, 98
Adipose deposits, types of 73
Adipose tissue 5, 6, 73, 109
   depots, perivascular 74
   distribution 6, 51, 89
      abnormal 6
   endocrine role of 84*t*
   involvement 6
   paradigm of 85
   perivascular 76
   role of 80-82
Adipsin 77
Adrenal
   adenomas 53
   androgens
      effect of 26
      secretes 20
   glands, physiology 20
   hormones 180
      precursor of 20
   insufficiency 26
   lipid content of 27
   medulla 27
   myelolipomas 53
   tumors, imaging of 27
Airway disease, obstructive 125
Alcoholism 124
Alirocumab 175, 177
Alpha-glucosidase inhibitors 155
American Diabetes Association 143
Amiodarone 125

Amphetamine-regulated transcript 80
Anabolic steroid 125
   misuse 6
Androgen 6, 155
   deprivation therapy 6, 156
Andropause 35, 36, 56
Androstenedione 20
Angiotensinogen 77
Antipsychotics 125
Apolipoprotein 12, 14, 36, 122, 123
Appetite 116
Aromatase 79
Arrhythmia 110
Artery disease, coronary 62, 99, 102, 102*t*
Asian lipophenotype 97, 98
   implications of 106*b*
   role of 100
Atherogenesis 61
Atherogenic dyslipidemia 47, 98
Atherosclerotic cardiovascular disease 51, 60-62, 65, 67, 103, 104, 172
   risk 62, 63, 104*fc*, 105
Atrial fibrillation 66
Atypical antipsychotic drugs 124
Autoimmune
   diabetes 52
   disorders 124, 125
Autosomal dominant 114

B

Barraquer-Simons syndrome 111
Berardinelli-Seip congenital lipodystrophy 114
Berardinelli-Seip syndrome 111
Beta-blockers 124, 125
Bile acid 12
   sequestrants 124, 143, 169
Birth weight 98
Blood pressure, high 103
Body frame 98
Body mass index 23, 51, 97, 98
Bone
   effects, clinical evidence of 166
   health 138
   marrow 74
      adipose tissue 76

metabolism 166
mineral density 7, 142, 166
morphometric protein 2 167
Bromocriptine 6
Brown adipose tissue 74, 75
distribution of 76f

C

Cabergoline 6
Calcium 163
channel blockers 165
Carbohydrate
intake, high 41
metabolism and diabetes 178
Carcinoma, hepatocellular 110
Cardiomyopathy 110
Cardiovascular disease 9, 65, 98, 100, 102, 104, 116, 160, 172
premature 41
Cardiovascular risk 24, 102
stratification 7, 55
Carotid intima media thickness 66, 148
Catecholamines 27
Cholesterol 123
acyltransferase 11
total 12, 14, 15, 52, 102, 122
Cholesteryl ester transfer protein 10, 11, 102, 149
Cholestyramine 7, 139, 140
role of 140t
Chylomicronemia, familial 41
Chylomicrons 61
Clofibrate 7, 140, 169
Clopidogrel 105
Clozapine 124
Co-existing disorders 164
Colchicine 165
Computed tomography 27, 53
Contrast-enhanced computed tomography 130
Cushing's syndrome 6, 7, 23-25, 28, 50, 51, 53, 64, 66, 67, 115, 126, 130, 131
management of 28, 152
Cushingoid habitus 6
Cyclophosphamide 124
Cyclosporine 124, 125, 165

D

Danazol 125
Dehydroepiandrosterone 20, 21, 32, 156
sulfate 21, 130
supplementation 156
Depomedroxyprogesterone 6
Diabetes 6, 7, 51, 53, 67, 83, 88, 125, 126, 128, 161
insipidus 7, 140

medications 153
mellitus 40, 74, 78, 87, 88, 98, 124, 142, 143
gestational 54
new-onset 161
pathogenesis of 87
risk of 178
Diacylglycerol 91
Diet and nutritional therapy 117
Dihydroepiandrosterone sulfate 141
Dipeptidyl peptidase-4 7, 79, 83, 142, 154
inhibitor 7, 154
Dopamine agonists 148
Drug therapy 105
concurrent 165
Dunnigan syndrome 111
Dysbetalipoproteinemia, familial 41, 123
Dysglycemia, combination of 98
Dyslipidemia 5-7, 19, 23, 24, 51, 56, 57, 60, 63, 66t, 98, 100, 103, 121, 122, 128t
combined 53, 122
diabetic 6
management of 25
secondary 124
types of 122, 124t
Dysphoria 37
Dysplasia, mandibuloacral 111

E

Endocrine
complications, management of 117
disease 7, 19, 54, 57, 63, 64, 64t, 66, 66t
diagnosis of 51
presence of 52
disorders 6, 7, 9, 56, 65, 121, 126t, 158
treatment of 7
drugs
effect of 6
lipid-lowering effects of 132
use of 6
dysfunction, mild 56
organ, secretes 6
vigilance 131
Endocrinology 1, 6, 50, 51, 53, 60
Endocrinopathy
diagnosis of 7
management of 137
Endoplasmic reticulum 90, 90f, 92
Endothelial dysfunction 91f
Energy homeostasis, regulator of 6
Enzymes 79t
Erectile dysfunction 7, 35, 55, 168
Erythromycin 165
Estrogen 6, 32, 41, 157
receptor 167
replacement therapy 35

treatment 157
Evolocumab 176, 177
Exocrine pancreas 39
Extracellular signal regulated kinase 166, 167
Ezetimibe 142

F

Farnesyl pyrophosphate 162, 167
Fasting plasma
   glucose 7
   triglyceride, abnormal 39
Fat distribution 6
Fatty acid
   nonesterified 63
   oxidation 44
   synthase 44
Fatty liver disease 93
   non-alcoholic 6, 7, 51, 73, 84, 116
Fenofibrate 138, 143, 169
Fibrates 125
Fibroblast growth factor 79, 84
Fluperlapine 124
Follicle-stimulating hormone 130
Framingham study 88
Frank obesity 98
Fredrickson's classification 123f
Free fatty acids 13, 36, 40, 43, 44, 75, 88, 90, 90f, 91, 92, 146
   effect of 92f
   receptor-1 92
   secretion, elevated 91f

G

Gallstone disease, absence of 41
Geranylgeranyl pyrophosphate 162, 167
Glomerulonephritis, membranoproliferative 114, 116
Glucagon, effect of 44
Glucagon-like peptide-1 154
   receptor agonists 7, 154
Glucocorticoids 6, 28, 41, 124, 125, 151
   chronic 23
   effect of 20, 21fc
   excess states 6
   increase lipolysis 63
   receptor 22
   reduce uncoupling protein 1 22
   regulate adipose tissue 21
   role of 25
   therapy 152
Glucose
   homeostasis 81, 116
   lowering drugs, effect of 179
   metabolism 178
   stimulated insulin secretion 45, 91

transporter-4 43, 81, 163
Glycemic
   control 7
   response 98
Glycerol phosphate 43
Gonadal development 33
Gonadal hormones 180
   effect of 32
Gonadopause 34
G-protein coupled receptor 40 91
Graves' disease 140, 140t
Growth 116
   factor, insulin-like 15, 66, 78, 130, 147
   hormone 6, 14, 16, 54, 63, 64, 66, 130, 146
      axis 146
      deficiency 6, 7, 16, 51, 57, 126, 129
      replacement therapy 148

H

Heart
   disease, coronary 10, 101, 122, 176
   failure 110
   protection study 142
Helsinki heart study 62
Hemorrhage, gastrointestinal 110
Hepatic
   insulin resistance 93
   lipase 149
   steatosis, metreleptin reduced 118
Hepatitis C virus 165
High triglyceride 124
   levels 62
High-density lipoprotein 7, 10, 11, 21, 23, 32, 36, 61, 64, 116, 125, 147, 149
   cholesterol 3, 7, 12-15, 24, 32, 47, 52, 102, 104, 122, 126, 139
   lower 62
   reduced 53, 99
Highly active antiretroviral therapy 110, 112
Hormonal therapy 37
Hormone 32, 146
   adrenocorticotropic 20, 130
   based therapies, lipid effects of 147t
   deficiency 6
   effect of 63
   luteinizing 130
   pancreatic 43f
   parathyroid 13
   regulate adipose tissue distribution and function 6
   regulate lipid metabolism 6
   replacement therapy 57
   sensitive lipase 44, 79
Human immunodeficiency virus 110, 114, 165
   associated lipodystrophy syndrome 112

infection 124, 125
Hydroxysteroid dehydrogenase 21, 79, 84
Hypercholesterolemia 172
    familial 6, 53, 123, 176
Hyperchylomicronemia, familial 123
Hyperglycemia, chronic 87
Hyperlipidemia 123*t*
    familial combined 41, 53, 123
Hyperlipoproteinemia 123
Hyperparathyroidism 55
    primary 14
    secondary 14
Hyperprolactinemia 53, 126, 129
Hypertension 83, 116
Hyperthyroidism 7, 14, 64, 66, 126, 128, 139
    effect of 13, 14*t*
    treatment of 151
Hypertriglyceridemia 39, 41, 53, 110, 125
    familial 41, 123
    induced acute pancreatitis 41*t*
        management of 41*t*
    mild-to-moderate 41
    moderate-to-severe 41
    severe 125
Hypogonadism 6, 7, 36, 53, 64, 66, 67, 126, 130
Hypoleptinemia 110
Hypoplasia, mandibular 116
Hypothalamic pituitary thyroid 151
Hypothyroidism 6, 7, 10, 12, 51, 53, 64, 66, 124-126, 128, 150
    effect of 12*b*, 12*t*
    subclinical 12, 64-66, 150

I

Indian Council of Medical Research India Diabetes Study 3, 122
Infection 125
Inflammation 82, 125
Insulin 6, 155
    effect of 43, 43*f*, 44
    receptor substrate 45
    resistance 7, 45, 91*f*, 98
    role of 44*t*
    secretion 91
    sensitivity 98, 116
Intracellular cholesterol transporter 13
Intramyocellular lipids 93
Ischemic disease 142
Isotretinoin 41, 125

K

Ketoconazole 6, 25, 132
Kidney
    disease, chronic 14, 53, 124, 125
    failure 110
Klinefelter's syndrome 36

L

Lactescent 41
L-asparaginase 124
Lawrence syndrome 111
Lecithin cholesterol acyltransferase 11, 13, 24, 64, 149, 151
Leptin 77
    deficiency 84
    receptors 80
Levothyroxine 150
Lipemia retinalis 41
Lipid
    abnormalities 10, 12, 42, 127*t*
    alteration 36, 64*t*
    disorders, management of 6
    metabolism 4, 61
    parameter 26, 64, 116
        serum 12, 14, 15
    profile, serum 52
    role of 31
    vigilance 7
Lipid-lowering
    agents 137
    drugs 7, 137, 161, 163, 164*t*, 166, 168
        endocrine effects of 7, 160, 161
    therapies 169, 172
Lipocalin 2 77
Lipocrinology 6, 7, 39, 43, 135
    definition and domains 3
    domains and scope 6*b*
    step toward newer insights 5
Lipodystrophy 7, 111, 114, 115, 115*b*, 118
    acquired generalized 111, 114, 114*t*, 116
    congenital generalized 111, 114, 116
    diagnosis of 115
    endocrine effects 109
    familial partial 111, 114, 116, 117
    HAART-induced 112
    hormonal and other manifestations of 116*t*
    inherited 110
    insulin-induced 111
    management of 116
    syndromes 110
    types 110
Lipogenesis 22
Lipo-health and endocrine system 9, 19, 30, 38
Lipolysis 22
Lipoprotein 7, 12, 14, 15, 61, 63, 122
    A 64
    cholesterol 89
    elevated 99
    intermediate-density 11, 13, 61, 123, 149
    lipase 11, 36, 44, 79
    metabolism 149*f*
Lipotoxicity 7, 46, 87, 90, 91, 93
Lipotropic considerations 146, 148

Index

Liver
  disease 110
    obstructive 125
  failure 110
Low fat intake 125
Low-density lipoprotein 7, 11, 21, 32, 44, 36, 61, 64, 113, 123, 125, 147, 149, 163, 174
  cholesterol 3, 7, 12, 14, 15, 23, 52, 105, 122, 126, 172
    elevated 53, 62, 99
  hepatic 146
  oxidized 11, 149
  receptor 10, 44, 162, 175

M

Macrolide antibiotics 165
Macroscopic fat 53
Magnetic resonance imaging 27, 53
Maturity-onset diabetes 52
Menarche, early 35
Menopause 34, 36, 125
Metabolic syndrome 6, 53, 56, 67, 82, 124, 142
Metformin 6, 117, 153
Metreleptin 118
Metyrapone 25
Mineralocorticoid
  effect of 26
  receptor 152
Mitogen activated protein kinase 167
Mitotane 25
Monitor endocrine therapy 7
Monocyte chemoattractant protein-1 75
Muscle
  insulin resistance 93
  syndromes 164t
  volume 98
Myalgia 164
Myocardial infarction 110
Myonecrosis 164
Myopathy 163-165
Myositis 164

N

Nasojejunal enteral feeding 40
National Cholesterol Education Program 98, 123
National Health and Nutrition Examination Survey 100
National Lipid Association Statin Muscle Safety Task Force 164t
Nephrotic syndrome 124, 125
Neuropathy, diabetic peripheral 143
Niacin 169
Niemann-Pick C1-like protein 1 173
Nitric oxide 163

Nucleoside reverse transcriptase inhibitors 113, 114

O

Obesity 6, 7, 25, 67, 82, 88, 125
  central 74
  visceral 6
Octreotide 6
Olanzapine 124
Omentin 78
Oral contraceptives 6
Oral estrogens 124
Organ, endocrine 5, 73
Osteoblast 166
  apoptosis 166
Osteoclastogenesis 166
Osteogenesis 166
Osteoprotegerin 167
Ovarian
  failure, premature 55
  insufficiency, premature 64, 66

P

Pancreas 38, 47
  endocrine 43
Pancreatic enzyme replacement therapy 42
Pancreatitis 116
  acute 39, 41, 110
  chronic 42
Paraproteinemias 125
Parathyroidectomy 14
Parenteral nutrition, total 40
Peroxisome proliferator-activated
  receptor 84
  alpha 4, 109, 138
  gamma 75, 80, 94, 153
Phosphatase 31
Phosphatidylinositol 3-kinase 90
Pituitary-growth hormone 179
Plasminogen activator inhibitor 1 75, 79, 82
Polycystic ovary
  disease 124, 125
  syndrome 6, 36, 51, 64-66, 73, 84, 110, 116, 126, 129, 138, 141
Polypeptide, pancreatic 38
Progesterone 32, 157
Progestin 125
Progranulin 78
Prolactin 16, 64, 148
Prolactinoma 64, 66
Propofol 41
Proprotein convertase subtilisin/kexin 9 10, 11, 26, 64, 174, 175, 179
  effect of 178
  inhibitors 7, 172, 173, 175t, 178

endocrine effects of 177
mechanism of action of 174f
pharmacodynamics of 177
pharmacokinetics of 177
Protease inhibitors 41, 113, 124
Puberty 6, 33, 81, 116, 125
precocious 35, 36

R

Raloxifene 124
Reactant protein secretion, acute phase 90f
Reactive oxygen species 90
Renin-angiotensin system 77
Reproduction 32fc
Reproductive
disorders 35, 36t
dysfunction 116
hormones, physiological actions of 32t
physiology 31
system 30
Resistin 78
Retinoids 124
Retinol binding protein 4 78, 79, 82
Retinopathy 139
diabetic 7, 138
Rhabdomyolysis, clinical 164
Ritonavir 165
Rosiglitazone 124

S

Saroglitazar 6
Scavenger receptor b-1 36
Sclerosis, amyotrophic lateral 164
Several genome-wide association studies 99
Sex chromosomal disorders 36
Sexual differentiation, disorders of 33
Sirolimus 124
Sodium-glucose co-transporter 2 inhibitors 154
Statin-associated myopathy 165t
Steatohepatitis, non-alcoholic 118
Steatorrhea 26
Steatosis, hepatic 110
Steroid
biosynthesis pathway 21fc
hormogenesis 168
sulfatase 79
Steroidogenic acute regulatory protein 20
Sterol regulatory element binding protein 2 11, 149, 174
Subcutaneous fat 6
Sulfonylureas 155
Syndrome of inappropriate antidiuretic hormone secretion 7

T

Tamoxifen 41, 124

Tensin homolog proteins 31
Testosterone 6, 32, 37
replacement therapy 156
Thermogenesis 80
Thiazide diuretics 124, 125
Thiazolidinedione 47, 125, 133, 153
Thyroid 149
disorders 65
hormone 6, 10, 11, 11f, 16, 149f, 179
effect of 149f
receptors 132
responsive elements 149
stimulating hormone 10, 66, 150
storm 140
Thyroidectomy 140
Thyromimetics 6, 150, 169
Thyroxine
replacement therapy 150
serum 10
Toll-like receptor 91
Transforming growth factor beta 166, 167b
Transsexual disorders 37
Triglycerides 12-15, 23, 36, 123
elevated 99
Tri-iodothyronine 10
Tumor necrosis factor alpha 22, 78, 79, 80, 82, 84
Turner's syndrome 36
Typical lipid abnormalities 126t

U

Unstable angina 105

V

Valproic acid 41
Vascular cell adhesion molecule-1 78
Very low-density lipoprotein 11, 13, 21, 22, 36, 40, 44, 61, 64, 99, 1234, 146, 149
cholesterol 52, 122
Visceral adipose tissue 74, 75t, 78
Vitamin D deficiency 42, 132, 165

W

Waist circumference 51, 98, 98t
Waist-hip ratio 98
White adipose tissue 74, 78

X

Xanthomas, eruptive 41

Z

Zona fasciculata 20
Zona glomerulosa 20
Zona reticularis 20